THE GLYCAEⁿ

THERESA CHEUNG is the
popular psychology books, inc~~luding~~ ~~....~~
All Evil, Get Lucky: Make Your Own Opportunities and
The Lazy Person's Guide to Stress. She also co-authored
the best-selling *PCOS Diet Book* and has contributed
features to *Here's Health, Health Plus, NHS Mother and
Baby, You Are What You Eat, Red, She* and *Prima*
magazines.

Overcoming Common Problems Series

Selected titles
A full list of titles is available from Sheldon Press,
36 Causton Street, London SW1P 4ST, and on our website at
www.sheldonpress.co.uk

Overcoming Common Problems Series

Coping with a Mid-life Crisis
Derek Milne

Coping with Polycystic Ovary Syndrome
Christine Craggs-Hinton

Coping with Postnatal Depression
Sandra L. Wheatley

Coping with SAD
Fiona Marshall and Peter Cheevers

Coping with Snoring and Sleep Apnoea
Jill Eckersley

Coping with a Stressed Nervous System
Dr Kenneth Hambly and Alice Muir

Coping with Strokes
Dr Tom Smith

Coping with Suicide
Maggie Helen

Coping with Thyroid Problems
Dr Joan Gomez

Depression
Dr Paul Hauck

Depression at Work
Vicky Maud

Depressive Illness
Dr Tim Cantopher

Eating for a Healthy Heart
Robert Povey, Jacqui Morrell and Rachel Povey

Effortless Exercise
Dr Caroline Shreeve

Fertility
Julie Reid

Free Your Life from Fear
Jenny Hare

Getting a Good Night's Sleep
Fiona Johnston

Heal the Hurt: How to Forgive and Move On
Dr Ann Macaskill

Heart Attacks – Prevent and Survive
Dr Tom Smith

Help Your Child Get Fit Not Fat
Jan Hurst and Sue Hubberstey

Helping Children Cope with Anxiety
Jill Eckersley

Helping Children Cope with Change and Loss
Rosemary Wells

Helping Children Get the Most from School
Sarah Lawson

How to Be Your Own Best Friend
Dr Paul Hauck

How to Beat Pain
Christine Craggs-Hinton

How to Cope with Bulimia
Dr Joan Gomez

How to Cope with Difficult People
Alan Houel and Christian Godefroy

How to Improve Your Confidence
Dr Kenneth Hambly

How to Keep Your Cholesterol in Check
Dr Robert Povey

How to Stick to a Diet
Deborah Steinberg and Dr Windy Dryden

How to Stop Worrying
Dr Frank Tallis

Hysterectomy
Suzie Hayman

Is HRT Right for You?
Dr Anne MacGregor

Letting Go of Anxiety and Depression
Dr Windy Dryden

Lifting Depression the Balanced Way
Dr Lindsay Corrie

Living with Alzheimer's Disease
Dr Tom Smith

Living with Asperger Syndrome
Dr Joan Gomez

Living with Asthma
Dr Robert Youngson

Living with Autism
Fiona Marshall

Living with Crohn's Disease
Dr Joan Gomez

Living with Diabetes
Dr Joan Gomez

Living with Fibromyalgia
Christine Craggs-Hinton

Living with Food Intolerance
Alex Gazzola

Living with Grief
Dr Tony Lake

Living with Heart Disease
Victor Marks, Dr Monica Lewis and Dr Gerald Lewis

Overcoming Common Problems Series

Overcoming Common Problems

The Glycaemic Factor
How to balance your blood sugar

Theresa Cheung

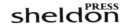

sheldon **PRESS**

First published in Great Britain in 2006

Sheldon Press
36 Causton Street
London SW1P 4ST

Copyright © Theresa Cheung 2006

British Library Cataloguing-in-Publication Data
A catalogue record for this book is available from the British Library

ISBN-13: 978–0–85969–975–4
ISBN-10: 0–85969–975–7

1 3 5 7 9 10 8 6 4 2

Typeset by Deltatype Ltd, Birkenhead, Wirral
Printed in Great Britain by
Ashford Colour Press

Contents

Introduction

If you want to beat food cravings, lose weight and enjoy optimal health, it's absolutely crucial to keep your blood sugar level steady. That in a nutshell is what this book is all about. There has been a great deal of media coverage in recent years of the glycaemic index (GI) as a way of eating that can promote both good health and weight loss. This book introduces the glycaemic load (GL) now known to be needed to complete the picture. Put simply, the GI measures foods according to how they affect blood sugar levels, both immediately and a few hours after a meal, while the GL looks at portion size, or how much you actually eat at a sitting.

Combining the GI with the GL helps you achieve a steady blood sugar level, without any highs or lows – which appears to be a key factor for weight management. A glycaemic diet is not complicated or time-consuming; it simply requires you to choose foods that will have a stabilizing effect on your blood sugar. Portion size and making sure you get all the nutrients you need for good health are the only things you need to be strict about. Eating the glycaemic way means that you don't feel hungry all the time and you don't need to weigh foods or count calories. You are encouraged to eat healthy fats and proteins and to avoid processed and refined foods. With its emphasis on whole grains, vegetables, fruits and legumes, the glycaemic diet works very well for vegetarians and vegans.

But this diet can also help a number of health conditions; it's not just about weight loss. It is valued by the medical profession, who approve of it because it's based on healthy eating plans, doesn't exclude vital foods, and isn't a crash diet. In fact, eating the glycaemic way has now become the new standard for healthy eating, healthy weight loss and healthy living.

This book offers a clear explanation of the GI and GL, referred to in the chapters that follow as the glycaemic factor, and the incredible health benefits a glycaemic factor diet has to offer – whether you want to lose weight, have a specific condition such as diabetes or polycystic ovary syndrome (PCOS) or want to undertake preventative healthcare and boost your health and wellbeing with a healthy eating plan.

It looks at the common misconceptions that exist about dieting and weight loss – such as the simple fallacy that eating less makes you automatically lose weight. It also explains why balancing your blood sugar can have such a range of health benefits, and how it may help with conditions such as obesity, premenstrual syndrome (PMS), PCOS, diabetes, high blood pressure, heart trouble, depression.

The book also gives practical tips to help you start and continue the diet, instructions on how to devise your own glycaemic factor eating plan, glycaemic factor tables for common foods, simple glycaemic factor meal plans, and rules for success.

Unlike fad diets, the glycaemic factor is based on science that you can follow for a lifetime. You'll discover a simple, delicious and satisfying formula for healthy eating that can not only help you lose weight and boost your energy levels but can also maximize your chances of optimum health, whatever your age!

1
What's all the fuss about?

For many years now, dieters have been searching for the philosopher's stone – a diet that can help them lose weight and keep it off, that doesn't require constant calorie counting and doesn't leave them feeling hungry. Could the glycaemic factor be the answer to every dieter's dream?

Here's a quick review of just some of the many popular diet plans in the last few years:

- The restrictive short-term diet plans, such as the Cabbage Soup Diet or the Beverly Hills Diet, suggest you eat one particular type of food and very little else. The downside, apart from the obvious vitamin and mineral deficiencies when you exclude variety from your diet, is that this kind of diet is incredibly hard to stick to.
- Meal replacement plans substitute vanilla and chocolate milk-shakes and nutrient bars for meals. The problem with this is that the bars and shakes, however much the advertisers describe them as 'delicious', can be bland and unsatisfying.
- Dr Atkins introduced his revolutionary new diet theory in the early 1970s. According to Atkins, if you cut out carbohydrates, such as bread, pasta and most fruits and vegetables, and focus on high fat proteins like meat and cheese instead, you'll lose weight. The idea is that cutting carbohydrates so radically forces your body to burn fat for fuel instead. People can and do lose weight on high protein diets, but they can also suffer from bad breath, headaches, constipation and fatigue as well as the threat of more serious health disorders such as kidney problems. Atkins-style or low carbohydrate diets remain popular in the twenty-first century despite the fact that most of the medical establishment is against a diet that restricts foods considered essential to health, such as fruits and whole grains. There have also been a number of well-publicized cases when dieters suffered severe metabolic disturbances and poor health as a result of the diet.
- Another diet to hit the scene in the 1970s was the Scarsdale Diet, which divided carbohydrates, proteins and fats into certain percentages. The diet lasts for 14 days with strict menu plans. The lack of calories is why most people lose weight in the short term

1

but in the long term weight tends to pile straight back on again, as it always does when weight is lost rapidly with severe calorie restriction. The Scarsdale is also, like the Atkins, high in protein, which means it can be very easy to consume an unhealthy amount of fat.

- The F-Plan Diet came next and the focus turned to the amount of fibre at every meal. Weight could be lost but the price paid was often digestive problems, stomach upsets, bloating and flatulence.

- Food combining diets appeared soon after. Rather than restrict either proteins or carbohydrates from your diet, food combining advocates say you can still eat both – just not at the same time. It's argued that different food groups digest at different rates so it's better for your digestion and metabolic rate to eat them separately. The downside with food combining is that the theory behind it simply hasn't got enough solid scientific backing yet for scientists, nutritionists and doctors to endorse it fully.

- The 1980s and 1990s were the Rosemary Conley decades as far as diets for weight loss were concerned. Conley books and videos sold millions all over the world, and continue to sell steadily today. The Conley diet plan is sensible and practical, but the emphasis on cutting right back on fat means that food often isn't that flavoursome and dieters can get very hungry between meals.

- From the early 1990s onwards new diets appeared constantly. Some of them focused on the drawbacks of previous diet plans while others suggested a unique approach of their own. For example, one plan suggests a diet according to your blood type, arguing that each blood type processes food differently. The Chocolate Diet divides chocoholics into six types and a diet is allocated to cope with their particular issues. The Omega Diet is based on a 12-food unit eating system to ensure an adequate intake of essential fats. The Schwarbein Principle Diet suggests that food be thought of in terms of how it affects your hormones. The Zone Diet is based on a ratio of at least 1:1 carbohydrates to protein at every meal, though this can go up to 2:1. There have also been trends that focus on ancient eating plans such as macrobiotics and ayurveda.

- As well as the many mainstream diets in every decade there have also been countless fad diets, such as the Cave Man Diet, the Russian Air Force Diet, the South Beach Diet, and so on. Fad diets sometimes produce short-term results, but no matter how clever, sophisticated and convincing a fad diet sounds, the great majority operate on one doomed ill-fated tactic: drastic calorie reduction. These doomed diets are hard to stick to, deprive the body of essential nutrients, trigger overeating due to deprivation and more often than not make it difficult to keep weight off in the long term. Many people who go on drastic fad diets find that even if they do successfully manage to lose weight it piles back on again as soon as they try to eat normally.

These are just some of the most well-known diet trends that have had their moment in the spotlight in recent decades, but none of them has completely fulfilled the dieter's dream of a satisfying diet that boosts energy and keeps weight off in the long term. Despite a wealth of diet options dieters still couldn't find the answer, but all this changed when the glycaemic index exploded on the diet and health scene in the late 1990s.

Everyone's talking about the glycaemic index

It might be a slight exaggeration to say everyone is talking about it, but judging by book sales millions of people are thinking about it.

Chapter 2 will explain this in more detail but, in brief, the glycaemic index (GI) is a ranking of foods based on their immediate effect on blood sugar levels. Carbohydrate foods that break down quickly during digestion have a high glycaemic value because their blood sugar response is fast and high. Carbohydrate foods that digest slowly and release glucose gradually into the bloodstream have low glycaemic values. Overconsumption of foods with a high glycaemic value can trigger insulin resistance and diabetes, as well as weight gain and other common health problems, all of which result from the long-term effects of too much insulin in the body.

Although it was originally devised for diabetes, where maintaining a steady blood sugar level is absolutely crucial, nutritionists began to appreciate how helpful the glycaemic index could also be for people who wanted to lose weight. Many of the diet bestsellers of recent years made recommendations based on the principle behind the GI – variations in the way different foods raise blood sugar and stimulate insulin – even though not all of them specifically used the glycaemic index as a tool. But it was Jennie Brand-Miller, PhD, from the University of Sydney, and her co-authors in *The Glucose Revolution: The Authoritative Guide to the Glycaemic Index,* published for the first time in the United States in 1999, which really focused public attention on the glycaemic index as a healthy eating guide for the nondiabetic as well as the diabetic.

The concept of a low glycaemic approach as a healthier and less restrictive diet than the typical high fat, low carbohydrate (carb), high protein regime had been around for 20 or so years previously but due to recent research[1] and recommendations from Harvard University it has finally began to reach the mainstream. As such dieticians, diabetic organizations and doctors are now paying attention to this important scientific reference to gauge the body's response to the carbohydrates we consume. Numerous studies[2] have shown that it has positive implications not only for obesity but also for heart health, diabetes and cancer prevention.

The glycaemic index (GI) is now billed as a lifestyle rather than a diet, helping consumers lose weight and stay healthy at the same time. It has firmly established itself on the diet scene as a revolutionary foundation for a lifetime of healthy eating that can also encourage weight loss. Despite all the hype, however, the GI diet does have certain limitations and restrictions.

Introducing the glycaemic load

What the GI doesn't tell you is how many carbohydrates are in a serving. This presents a problem. You might be tempted, for example, to eliminate a food like carrots from your diet due to their extremely high GI value even though carrots are a nutritious and healthy food choice. That's where the glycaemic load (GL), which is explained in detail in Chapter 3, comes in. The GL takes into consideration a food's GI as well as the amount of carbohydrates per serving, which means that nutritious foods, like carrots, don't need to be eliminated.

The GL is the next step on from the GI diets. Research[3] suggests that using it as a guide to food choices is one of the healthiest ways to make the long-term changes needed to achieve and maintain a healthy weight, reduce the risk of health problems related to poor nutrition, and get all the nutrients you need from a well-balanced diet. It offers a wide range of choices without calorie counting or restriction and, best of all, offers freedom from hunger and cravings.

'Though the glycaemic index of a food is helpful information, it is only part of the story. The glycaemic load (GL) better reflects a food's effect on your body's biochemistry than either the amount of carbohydrates or the glycaemic index alone.' (Dr Walter Willett, MD Dr PH, Chairman of the Department of Nutrition at the Harvard School of Public Health and Professor of Medicine at Harvard Medical School.)

The glycaemic factor is here to stay

Combining the GI with the GL, which in this book for simplicity is referred to as the glycaemic factor, could finally end the search for an eating plan that helps you lose or maintain your weight without sacrificing your health in the process. In Chapter 4 you'll discover why and how the glycaemic factor can help you manage your weight, and in Chapter 5 you'll discover the other incredible health benefits it offers. The remaining chapters of the book outline how the glycaemic factor can be easily incorporated into a healthy eating plan that works for all the family. There are also reference tables, meal plans and motivational tips to get you started.

Without a doubt the glycaemic factor is here to stay. It's not a fad diet. It's a tool for healthy eating, weight loss and optimum health that, unlike previous trends in dieting, actually has the backing and blessing of medical research behind it. And if you're looking for a compact guide to the glycaemic factor that is designed to help you establish a healthy weight and a healthier way of eating for a lifetime – no matter what your age, sex, weight or physical condition – this book has been written for you.

2

What you need to know about the glycaemic index

Since the 1980s, scientific research into the glycaemic index clearly demonstrates that a number of common beliefs about food, carbohydrates, weight loss and health that we hold today are simply not true. For example:

- *Belief: sugar is fattening.*
  Just because a food is high in sugar does not necessarily mean it is fattening. Sugar is not more likely to be turned into fat than any other carbohydrate. It is often present in foods with concentrated energy and fat, but it's the total calories rather than the sugar in these foods which cause more fat to be made. And while we are on the subject of sugar, let's dispel a couple of other myths: sugar does not cause high blood pressure (it's salt people with high blood pressure need to watch out for), sugar is not the worst thing for people with diabetes (fat can be most harmful) and a diet high in sugar is not always high in fat. In fact, diets high in fat are often low in sugar, and diets high in sugar are often low in fat.
- *Belief: hunger is a regrettable but inevitable part of losing weight.*
  Simply not true. If you're dieting and feeling hungry all the time you are more likely to gain rather than lose weight. The secret of weight loss is to keep your metabolism (calorie-burning) high with regular meals and snacks and to eat plenty of low GI foods that can satisfy your appetite until the next meal.
- *Belief: skipping breakfast can keep your calorie count and your weight down.*
  Not true. Overweight people miss breakfast. Eating a healthy, hearty breakfast gets your metabolism (calorie-burning) off to a flying start.
- *Belief: fattening foods are more filling.*
  Not true. Studies[4] show that foods high in fat are often the least filling.
- *Belief: if you want to lose weight you've got to stick to the same meal plans and menus.*
  Not true. Variety is the spice of life and it's also the key to the

6

success of any healthy eating plan. Varying your diet and eating lots of different foods ensures that you are getting all the nutrients you need to help you lose weight.

- *Belief: if you want to lose weight you need to cut down on fat.* Not true. It depends on the type of fat. Saturated fats and transfats found in animal products are fattening and unhealthy but essential fats such as omega 3 and omega 6, found in oily fish, nuts and seeds, can actually help you lose weight and should not be excluded from your diet.

- *Belief: if you want to lose weight, eat less.* Not true. Eating less or fasting will not help you lose weight in the long term. One of the most effective ways to lose weight is to eat more rather than less as long as the foods you eat are nutrient rich and have a stabilizing effect on your blood sugar.

- *Belief: if you want to lose weight you need to cut down on carbohydrates.* Not true. You may lose weight on a low carbohydrate diet but it is a diet that is very hard to stick to and as soon as you eat normally again the weight will pile back on. Contrary to popular belief that low carbohydrate diets are the best way to lose weight, research[5] indicates that the right amount of the right kind of carbohydrate can not only help you lose weight but also boost your health and wellbeing. This is because the right kinds of carbohydrates play a key role in maintaining steady blood sugar levels and, as we'll explore below, a steady blood sugar level, without any highs or lows, appears to be a key factor for weight management.

- *Belief: the best way to lose weight is to eat a low calorie diet.* Calories are one of the contributing factors in weight gain but certainly not the whole story. What a calorie-controlled diet doesn't take into account is the fat-storing ability of specific carbohydrates due to their effect on blood sugar levels. Balancing blood sugar levels has been shown to be crucial when it comes to weight loss and good health. When we eat high glycaemic foods (ones that deliver sugar quickly to the bloodstream) we have a rapid increase in glucose which prompts a rapid release in insulin (one of the most powerful hormones in the body) to clear the glucose out of the bloodstream into the liver and muscles where it is stored for later use. But if we constantly eat high glycaemic foods, even those that are low in calories and fat, this leads to overproduction of insulin and storage of glucose in our fat cells, which is why we put on weight. Balancing blood sugar levels, not calorie counting, is the best way to lose weight.

Why we need to keep blood sugar levels steady

All our cells get their energy from a steady supply of sugar in our blood. To stay healthy, we need to control the amount of sugar in our blood because, apart from not functioning at our best, sharp fluctuations in blood sugar levels are undesirable to our general health. Medical experts[6] unanimously agree that fluctuating blood sugar levels increase the risk of developing obesity, diabetes, high blood fat levels, high blood pressure and heart disease.

Insulin is the hormone that regulates your blood sugar levels. It breaks down sugar and delivers energy in the form of glucose and fat to your body's cells. Every time you eat food, the pancreas gland excretes insulin. In a balanced state your bloodstream contains about two teaspoons of glucose. When this amount is exceeded, by eating carbohydrates with a high glycaemic value, your body produces large amounts of insulin to mop up the excess glucose to bring blood sugar levels down. Once blood sugar levels have come down, the sharp drop can trigger cravings, fatigue and mood swings. Also, the blood sugar your body doesn't use as fuel is stored as body fat by insulin, increasing the likelihood of weight gain.

In short, too much insulin in your bloodstream can become a health problem and increase the likelihood of fatigue, overeating and weight gain. Insulin also stops dieters from feeling the cut-off point after a meal that tells them they have had enough, so if your insulin levels are high you are more likely to overeat. The key to good health is therefore to stabilize blood sugar over a sustained period of time and to avoid the roller-coaster of highs and lows which trigger sharp rises in insulin followed by storage of excess sugar as fat.

The importance of maintaining steady blood sugar levels is something, of course, that diabetics and people who are insulin resistant have known about for a long time.

Regulating blood sugar levels

If you eat foods that trigger the release of too much insulin over a long period of time, as in months and years, your body's cells become resistant to the insulin. Insulin resistance is a medical term that means the body's cells do not respond properly to insulin. They don't uptake glucose and fat properly and there is too much insulin in the bloodstream. This leads to weight gain and an increased risk of type 2 diabetes.

If you are a person with type 2 diabetes or insulin resistance or impaired glucose tolerance, also known as borderline diabetes, your body has problems uptaking blood sugar into the cells; it can't use insulin efficiently any more and consequently your blood sugar levels stay too high. Elevated blood sugar levels can lead to damaged blood vessels, eye disease, heart disease, early dementia, nerve damage to the limbs and internal organs and kidney disease. In addition, diabetics often continue to gain weight, leading to obesity, which has its own set of health risks.

Diabetics and people with blood sugar disorders have to be very careful about their sugar intake, and part of their treatment plan is to focus on foods that provide slow, steady amounts of energy throughout the day to avoid rapid rises in blood sugar. Research[7] has shown that blood glucose levels after a meal are most affected by the amount of carbohydrates eaten – but not all carbohydrates, starches and sugar produce blood sugar swings because some are broken down more steadily and slowly in the digestive system. In the 1980s, scientists began to test different types of carbohydrates and give each a score according to how quickly they converted into blood sugar. This score became known as the glycaemic index, from the term 'glycogen', the form in which sugars are stored in the body.

It's easy to see why the glycaemic index has become an invaluable tool for the treatment of diabetics and blood sugar disorders. It can help diabetics plan meals that will stabilize their blood sugar and insulin levels and so help them manage their condition.

The glycaemic index

The glycaemic index was developed by David Jenkins and his team of scientists at the University of Toronto in 1981 to express the rise of blood sugar (glucose) after eating a particular carbohydrate, and it soon replaced the older method of classifying carbohydrates according to their simple or complex structure.

The index compares the blood sugar response to a particular food with the body's reaction to pure glucose, which is given the value of 100, the top score. For example, if a food raises blood sugar only half as much as pure glucose, that food is given a glycaemic index of 50. The portion size used to test the glycaemic index of various foods is the amount that contains 50 grams of carbohydrate. Some research has used white bread instead of glucose as the standard of comparison for determining the glycaemic index of foods. The glycaemic index of a food is governed by several factors, such as the form of carbohydrate it contains, the amount and form of fibre it contains, how much processing and cooking it has been subjected to, and the presence of other substances such as protein and fat.

In the glycaemic index, carbohydrates are classified into three main groups – high, medium and low – according to how quickly they are turned into blood sugar by the body. The higher a food appears on the index, the faster it induces insulin and therefore the greater its undesirability. The lower a food's GI the more slowly the food will convert into blood sugar, promoting a weaker insulin response.

The underlying premise for advocating eating low glycaemic index foods is that high glycaemic index foods cause a rapid elevation in blood sugar that the body attempts to balance by producing a large amount of insulin. Advocates claim that human physiology is not designed to tolerate these rapid and prolonged elevations in blood sugar and insulin caused by the prevalence of modern, high glycaemic index foods in the diet. As human civilization has evolved, primitive Stone Age diets that featured naturally occurring, low carbohydrate foods have been replaced, first by unprocessed but higher carbohydrate agricultural foods such as whole grains and legumes, and more recently by highly processed, low fibre flours and other starchy foods, plus an increasing amount of sweets. This trend towards higher glycaemic index foods in the diet is therefore deemed unnatural and a threat to the healthy functioning of the body.

As we've seen, overproduction of insulin can lead to insulin resistance, in which cells that normally respond to insulin become less sensitive to its effects. Excessive consumption of high GI foods can trigger blood sugar problems and high insulin levels and by so doing increase the risk of obesity, type 2 diabetes, heart disease and some cancers. Changing to a low GI diet has been shown in many studies[8] to reduce insulin resistance, help control appetite, improve weight loss results, enhance blood sugar control in diabetics, lower cholesterol and reduce the risk of heart disease.

How do people use the GI?

People use the GI to help them choose carbohydrate-containing foods that will only minimally raise their blood sugar levels, with the intent of preventing health problems associated with either high blood sugar or the body's reaction to rising blood sugar. Foods with a GI of 55 and below are considered ideal for those trying to consume low GI foods.

High GI foods such as white bread, chips and doughnuts score between 70 and 100. Medium GI foods, scoring between 55 and 70, include bran and fruit cereals and figs; low GI foods score less than 55 and include grapefruit, plain yogurt and red kidney beans.

Do bear in mind that every person will have a slightly different insulin response to each food, but typically when you eat a high GI food, you get an immediate rush of energy because of the high blood sugar levels. The resulting insulin response removes the sugar from your blood, so you now begin to feel fatigued. Eating foods low on the GI will keep you from going through this roller-coaster of high and low blood sugar. Your blood sugar levels will remain more level throughout the day, which will give you a feeling of high energy all day long.

The GI of foods can vary considerably. Cooking, especially overcooking, foods will increase their GI. Below is a partial list of the GI of some common foods. This list uses glucose as the standard and has a rating of 100. You'll find a fuller and more detailed listing of GI food ratings online at: <www.glycaemicindex.com>.

Breads

White bread	96
Waffle	76
Doughnut	76
Wholewheat bread	75
Bread stuffing	74
Kaiser rolls	73
Bagel, white	72
Melba toast	70
Tortilla, corn	70
Rye bread	65
Wholewheat pitta	58
Pumpernickel bread	49

Cereals

Puffed Rice	90
Cornflakes	84
Rice Krispies	82
Coco Pops	77

Cheerios	74
Shredded Wheat	69
Puffed Wheat	67
Grape-Nuts	67
Muesli	66
Porridge	55
Special K	54
All Bran	42

Crackers/biscuits

Vanilla wafers	77
Rice cakes	92
Water crackers	72
Golden Grahams	71
Shortbread	64

Dairy products

Ice cream	61
Pizza cheese	60
Ice cream – low fat	50
Milk – skimmed	32
Yogurt – with sugar	33
Yogurt – no sugar	14

Fruits

Watermelon	72
Dried fruit	70
Pineapple	66
Cantaloupe	65
Blueberry	59
Orange juice	57
Mango	55
Fruit cocktail	55
Banana	53
Kiwi	52
Orange	43
Grapes	43
Pear	35
Apple	35
Strawberry	32
Grapefruit	25

Plum	25
Cherries	23
Raisins	64

Grains

Rice – instant	88
Millet	71
Rice – white/not instant	70
Cornmeal	68
Rye flour	65
Couscous	65
Bran	60
Buckwheat	54
Bulgar	48
Barley, pearled	25

Legumes

Fava beans	80
Baked beans – canned	68
Romano beans	46
Black-eyed peas	42
Chick peas	33
Split peas	32
Lima beans – frozen	32
Butter beans	31
Black beans	30
Lentils	29
Beans – dried	29
Kidney beans	27
Soya beans	18

Pasta

Brown rice pasta	92
Refined pasta	65
Gnocchi	65
Wholegrain – thick	45
Angel hair	45
Star pastina	38
Wholegrain spaghetti	37
Vermicelli	35

13

Vegetables

Parsnips	97
Potato – baked	85
Potato – instant	83
Pumpkin	75
Chips	75
Potato – fresh, mashed	73
Rutabaga (a sort of turnip)	72
Carrot	71
Beets	64
New potatoes	62
Sweetcorn	55
Sweet potato	54
Yam	51
Tomato	38
Green vegetables	low
Bean sprouts	low
Cauliflower	low
Eggplant	low
Peppers	low
Squash	low
Onions	low
Water chestnuts	low

Miscellaneous

Glucose	100
Rice cake	82
Jelly beans	80
Pretzels	80
Honey	73
Corn chips	73
Soft drink	70
Sucrose	65
Hamburger bun	61
Sponge cake	54
Chocolate	49
Instant noodles	47
Fructose	23

One of the best ways to put the GI theory into practice is to substitute, wherever possible, low GI foods for high GI foods, to lower the overall glycaemic index of your diet. For example:

- High GI bread (white or wholewheat) can be replaced by the low GI alternative of whole grains, stoneground flour bread and breads that don't contain enriched wheat flour.
- High GI rice (short grain, quick-cooking brown or white rice) can be replaced by long grain white and brown rice and basmati.
- High GI baked potatoes and instant mash can be replaced by sweet potatoes, yams and new potatoes.
- Pasta and noodles that are overcooked can be replaced by pasta and noodles cooked al dente.
- Gluten-free corn and millet can be replaced by barley and buckwheat.
- Processed breakfast cereals can be replaced by granola, rolled oats, Grape-Nuts, Special K, muesli and oat bran.
- When choosing fruit opt for apples, pears, citrus fruits, cherries, peaches and plums in preference to mango, pineapple, dates, watermelon and raisins.
- When choosing crackers opt for Ryvita and stoneground wheat thins rather than rice cakes and other types of cracker.
- When it comes to legumes (beans, chickpeas, lentils) eat as much of them as you like as all legumes are low GI.

How to tell if a food has a low, medium or high GI value

Without a book or a table at hand it isn't always easy to tell if a food has a high, medium or low GI. In the science laboratories GI testing can take hours. Each volunteer is given a carefully measured portion of the food to be tested that is known to contain 50g of carbohydrate. Blood tests are then taken every 15 minutes for the first hour and every 30 minutes for the second hour and blood sugar level is charted. The volunteer's response to the food is then compared to their response to consuming 50g of glucose, the reference food. The reference and test food scores are compared for ten subjects and the food is finally awarded a GI score.

Clearly this isn't the kind of test you can do at home so here are some basic guidelines.

It's not necessary to avoid high GI foods completely. When these foods are combined in a meal with low GI foods or with certain proteins and fats then the overall glycaemic effect is reduced. Of course, to lower the overall glycaemic index of the diet, low GI foods should be emphasized as much as possible.

The basic rules are to reduce your intake of concentrated sugars and increase your consumption of fresh foods such as legumes and most vegetables and fruits, and choose grain products made by traditional methods (for example, pasta, stoneground flour products, old-fashioned porridge) rather than those produced with modern technology (highly refined flour products, low fibre flaked breakfast cereals, quick-cooking starches, etc.)

Perhaps the simplest way to distinguish between easily absorbed carbohydrates and more slowly absorbed ones is by taste. As a rule of thumb, the sweeter the taste, the quicker you're going to get a blood sugar rush. Obviously simple sugars are the fastest to be converted, and you'll find them listed on food labels with names such as glucose, sucrose, dextrose and maltose. Refined processed carbohydrates are quick to convert because they lack fibre, but wholegrains, seeds, beans and legumes and some vegetables contain a high percentage of dietary fibre which slows down their digestion. The lower the fibre content of a certain food, the higher its GI is likely to be.

As a quick guide the following foods rank highest on the glycaemic index. (These foods should be avoided or kept to a minimum by those wishing to consume a low glycaemic index diet.)

- white rice;
- rice cakes;
- most breads, breakfast cereals, snacks and desserts made with refined flour products;
- potatoes (except new potatoes, sweet potatoes and yams).

Fats, oils, and sweets to avoid:

- soft drinks, including sweetened fruit drinks and most sports drinks;
- most cakes and pies;
- sweets and chocolate bars;
- granola bars and most sports bars;
- raisins;
- overripe bananas.

16

The following foods rank medium to low on the glycaemic index:

• whole grain breads;
• breads containing whole, intact grains and seeds (millet, flaxseed, etc.);
• brown rice, basmati rice;
• barley, buckwheat;
• wholegrain cereals, muesli;
• wholewheat pitta, chapatis;
• porridge;
• legumes and legume products (hummus, baked beans, lentil soup, etc.);
• bakery products made with whole grains, bran, whole fruit pieces, and/or nuts;
• unsweetened milk and milk products;
• unsweetened yogurt;
• soya beverages.

Most vegetables and vegetable juices and many fruits have low GIs. The following have such a low GI that they can be eaten as often as you want, especially in their raw form:

• apples;
• cabbage;
• celery;
• cherries;
• cucumber;
• lettuce;
• parsley;
• peaches;
• pears;
• plums;
• radishes;
• spinach;
• turnips;
• watercress.

Are there any cons to the GI diet?

Critics say that the way the glycaemic index is measured (one food at a time in quantities that contain a standard amount of carbohydrate) does not resemble the way people usually eat (many items are

eaten together in varying portion sizes, often mixing high carbohydrate with low carbohydrate foods). It also only measures the short-
term and not the long-term effect. Not to mention the fact that
certain foods that are high in the glycaemic index, such as carrots,
are nutritional superstars that should not be excluded from a healthy
diet.

In answer to these criticisms, advocates point to the many studies[9]
linking diets containing high glycaemic index foods to common and
serious health problems. They insist that the diet can take into
account portion size and include high glycaemic, nutrient-rich foods,
such as carrots, by combining the glycaemic index with the
glycaemic load, a concept we'll explore in more detail in the next
chapter. They also insist that the diet can be made more healthful by
integrating it with other health concepts, such as those listed below,
to achieve the best results.

GI diet recommendations

You won't automatically lose weight if you consume an excessive
amount of low GI foods or foods that aren't carbohydrates. Diets
that focus on the GI as a healthy eating tool also recommend a
sensible balance of nutrients obtained from all three food groups –
carbohydrates, proteins and fats – to ensure your body is getting
everything it needs for good health.

On a GI diet it is typically suggested that you consume around
five to eight servings a day of fruit and vegetables. You should also
consume between three and eight servings of carbohydrates, between
one and three servings of meat, poultry, fish, eggs, beans and nuts
and between one and three servings of low fat milk, yogurt and
cheese. Fats, oils and sugary treats should only be eaten rarely.

Protein and fat

Although only carbohydrates are given a GI value on a GI diet, an
adequate intake of healthy fat and protein is also essential to ensure
you are getting all the nutrients you need for weight management
and good health. Proteins are crucial for good health and provide the
amino acids from which bones, muscles, hair, nails, blood, hormones
and brain chemicals are made. They also help maintain blood sugar
balance and give your body an even supply of energy. Since your

body can't store amino acids, as it does carbohydrate and fat, you need a constant, daily supply of them.

Contrary to popular opinion, proteins aren't just found in meat and dairy products; you can find them in vegetables, whole grains such as quinoa, soya products like tofu, beans and pulses, nuts, seeds, brown rice, broccoli, bananas and other fruits and vegetables.

In addition to carbohydrate and protein you also need some fat in your diet, even if you are trying to lose weight. You should try to obtain as little fat as possible from saturated fats found in many animal food sources and commercial foods, such as biscuits and snacks, and hydrogenated or transfats found in various kinds of ready meals, biscuits, cakes, breads and spreads, vegetable shortening, peanut butter, pastries, margarines and fast foods. Saturated and trans fatty acids have been associated with an increased risk of weight gain and high levels of cholesterol, blocking the arteries and triggering heart disease and strokes. Instead you should try to obtain as much fat as possible in the form of monosaturated fats found in olive oil and essential fatty acids, such as omega 3 and omega 6 fatty acids, found in oily fish like salmon, mackerel and herring, flaxseed oils, wheat germ, nuts, seeds, vegetable oils and soya beans. Your body needs essential fats to regulate hormone function, thin the blood and strengthen cell walls. What's more, high quality fat also slows down the entry of carbohydrates to the system thus keeping insulin levels lower. In fact, dietary fats are one of the best blood sugar stabilizers.

Vitamins and minerals

Unlike high protein, low carbohydrate diets, the GI diet doesn't expect you to cut out or restrict any food group. An adequate and balanced intake of not only carbohydrate but also protein and fat is emphasized because if you're eating a balanced diet, this means you are more likely to get all the vitamins and minerals you need for good health.

Below are listed the key vitamins and minerals, their functions and the foods they can be found in. It's important to eat foods containing these important nutrients on a daily basis. If this isn't always possible a good insurance policy is to take a multivitamin and mineral supplement on a regular basis, as long as you remember that supplements cannot ever be a substitute for a healthy diet.

Vitamins

A vitamin is any group of organic substances – other than proteins, carbohydrates, fats, minerals and organic salts – which are essential for normal metabolism, growth, health and development. Vitamins regulate metabolic processes, control cellular functions and boost immunity.

Vitamin A

Essential for normal growth, strong bones, healthy skin and healing. Lack of Vitamin A can lead to infection of the cornea, conjunctiva (the red part of the eye), trachea (windpipe), hair follicles and renal system. Deficiency can also cause night blindness.

Vitamin A is found in butter, egg yolk, fish oils, liver, some fruits (prunes, pineapples, oranges, limes and cantaloupe), green leafy vegetables and carrots.

B vitamins

Vitamin B1 (thiamine) affects growth, appetite, nerve function and carbohydrate metabolism. B1 is found in whole grains, beans, nuts, egg yolk, fruits and most vegetables.

Vitamin B2 (riboflavin) affects growth and energy production. It is found in liver, meat, poultry, eggs and green vegetables.

Vitamin B3 (niacin) is essential for digestion, energy and the nervous system. It is found in meat, poultry, whole grains and peanuts.

Vitamin B5 (pantothenic acid) strengthens immunity, fights infections, heals wounds and helps counteract the negative effects of stress. It is found in fish, eggs, chicken, nuts and whole grains.

Vitamin B6 (pyridoxine) is essential for the production of new cells and a healthy immune system. It is found in meat, eggs, whole grains, yeast, cabbage and melon.

Vitamin B12 (cyanocobalamin) is needed for energy and concentration and growth in children. It is found in oily fish, meat, eggs, milk and wheat cereals.

Folic acid is essential for new cells and is especially important during pregnancy for the prevention of birth defects. It is found in fruit, green vegetables, nuts and pulses.

Vitamin C (ascorbic acid)

Necessary for healthy skin, bones, muscles, eyesight and protection against viruses. It is found in raw cabbage, carrots, orange juice, lettuce, celery, onions, tomatoes and all citrus fruits.

Vitamin D

Necessary for the development of bones and teeth. It is essential in the metabolism of calcium and phosphorus, two of the most important constituents of bones and teeth. Vitamin D is manufactured in the skin with exposure to sunlight, and is also found in milk, cod liver oil, salmon, egg yolk and butter fat.

Vitamin E

Essential for the absorption of iron and fatty acids, slowing the aging process and boosting fertility. It is found in nuts, seeds, whole grains, leafy vegetables, soya and avocados.

Vitamin K

Essential for blood clotting, Vitamin K is found in green vegetables, apricots and whole grains.

Minerals

Minerals are essential, acting as co-factors of enzymes (enzymes are the essential catalysts of all the chemical reactions in the body; without them we would cease to exist) and organizers of the molecular structure of the cell and its membrane.

Calcium

Needed for strong bones and teeth as well as hormones, muscles and the regulation of blood clotting. Good sources include leafy green vegetables, dairy produce, salmon, nuts, root vegetables and tofu.

Chromium

Necessary for the maintenance of normal blood sugar levels. Chromium works with insulin in assisting cells to take in glucose and release energy. Some good sources include whole grains, meat, brewer's yeast, egg yolk and mushrooms.

Copper

Needed for the production of red blood cells and the formation of connective tissues. Some sources include meat, seafood, nuts and seeds.

Fluorine

Maintains the structure of teeth. Sources include water (in some areas), seafood, kidney, liver and other meats.

Iron

Essential for oxidizing the cells and for boosting immunity. It is found in dark chocolate, shellfish, pulses, green leafy vegetables, egg yolk, beans and molasses.

Magnesium

Essential for the transmission of nerve impulses, development of bones, growth and repair of cells. It can be found in nuts, beans, whole grains and legumes.

Manganese

The activator of many enzymes. Manganese is very closely related to the synthesis of DNA, RNA and protein. Sources include whole grains and cereals, fruits and vegetables.

Potassium

Essential for maintaining water balance, nerve and muscle function. It is found in avocados, leafy green vegetables, bananas, fruit, potatoes, vegetable juices and nuts.

Selenium

Important in protecting lipids of cell membranes (cell walls are made up of a lipid (fat) layer), proteins and nucleic acids against oxidant damage. Sources include broccoli, chicken, cucumbers, egg yolk, garlic, liver, milk, mushrooms, onions, seafood and tuna. Brazil nuts are a rich source, but don't eat them more than three times a week; they are high in saturated fat.

Zinc

Essential for synthesis of protein, DNA and RNA. Required for growth in all stages of life and for healthy reproduction. Sources include meats, oysters and other seafood, milk and egg yolk.

One way to increase your chances of getting all the vitamins and minerals you need is to make sure the portions of vegetables and fruits you eat in a day are different colours: dark green spinach, yellow corn, red peppers, orange carrots, blackberries and so on. Make sure your plate is filled with the natural colours of fresh food and you will be getting your nutrients.

Reading food labels

It's important to pay attention to food labels and get used to spotting hidden ingredients. Although there are signs that supermarkets may start using low GI signs in the future, at present you are unlikely to find a low GI sign on food labels. You should, however, find that reading the list of ingredients on the food label while also bearing in mind the GI diet recommendations can help you decide if a food is high GI or low GI.

We are fortunate today that food manufacturers are required to list the ingredients in their products, but all too often food labels can be confusing and misleading for consumers. The following guidelines should make things easier for you.

From top to bottom

Ingredients are usually listed in descending order of volume so if sugar and fat are at the top of the list you know it's going to be high GI.

Long list of additives, preservatives, colourings, emulsifiers, stabilizers, thickeners and E numbers

Some chemicals are harmless – for instance, ammonium bicarbonate, malic acid, fumaric acid, lactic acid, lecithin, xanathan, guar gums, calcium chloride, monocalcium phosphate and monopotassium phosphate – but how can you tell when there is a long list of chemical names that look unfamiliar to you? If that's the case a good general rule is simply to avoid products whose chemical ingredients outnumber the familiar ones.

Long list of names you don't recognize

More and more manufacturers are cleaning up their products as people are becoming more concerned about healthy eating and you will increasingly see 'no artificial sweeteners' or 'no artificial ingredients'. This is helpful but watch out still for hidden fats, salts and sugars and alternative names for foods that aren't very good for you when eaten in excess. Sugar, for example, has lots of different names and they include: sucrose, fructose, dextrose, corn syrup, malt syrup, honey, galactose and maple syrup. Mannitol, sorbitol, xylitol, saccharine and aspartame are just alternative names for potentially carcinogenic artificial sweeteners. You'll probably recognize the names for fats. Steer clear of saturated fat, hydrogenated, partially hydrogenated, polyunsaturated and transfats. If you can't understand a label, though, or there's barely room for all the chemical ingredients, leave the product on the shelf.

Watch out for misleading claims

'No added sugar' or 'unsweetened' does not mean that a food is low in sugar; it simply means no sugar has been added during processing.

'Rich source of . . .' means that the product must contain 50 per cent of the recommended daily amount (RDA) in a suggested serving. If it says 'source of' it must contain 17 per cent.

The term 'fat free' means foods containing less than 0.15g fat per 100g. However, the term '80 per cent fat free' means the product actually has 20 per cent fat. 'Virtually fat free' means the food has less than 0.3g fat per 100g. 'Low fat' means that the food must contain less than 3g of fat per 100g. 'Reduced fat' means the food contains 25 per cent less fat than equivalent products.

Calorie count is typically given per portion, per pack and per 100g. Do remember that manufacturers' portion sizes can be extremely small, and whatever diet you are on, if you consume more calories a day than you burn off you will put on weight – even if these calories are low GI calories.

Some GI diet tips

Protein and fat can slow down the digestion of carbohydrate so you can use them to slow down the effects of a high GI food on your blood sugar. For example, a boiled egg on toast will have a far lower GI value than toast and jam.

Foods that are high in fibre tend to be lower GI than products that have had the fibre taken away. Apples are low GI but apple juice has a medium GI because the fibre has been removed. The same applies to wholegrain products versus refined white products.

- If you eat a low GI food with a high GI food this will balance things out to produce a medium GI food.
- The more natural and less processed the food is, the more likely it is to be low GI.
- Cooking can alter the GI value of food. The longer something is cooked the less nutrients and fibre will remain; lightly steaming or eating vegetables raw makes your digestive system work harder and lowers the GI value of the meal.
- Acids seem to be able to lower a food's GI value. For example, sprinkling vinegar or lemon juice on a meal can lower its overall GI.
- However many low GI foods you consume, you won't lose weight or feel healthier unless you also ensure that you are getting a sensible balance of nutrients and plenty of variety in your meals.
- Bear in mind that as helpful as the GI is when it comes to creating a healthy eating plan, it can still at times be misleading and confusing. This is because it doesn't take into account portion size. Another measure does, however, take portion size into account and that measure is called the *glycaemic load*.

3

Introducing the glycaemic load

The previous chapter explained how the glycaemic index (GI) can be used to help you choose low GI carbohydrates that can supply you with a steady, constant amount of energy and not produce an overload that will be stored as fat. The GI has limitations, though, as it does not take into account portion size. The glycaemic load (GL), on the other hand, does consider portion size. It's the final part of the jigsaw and the focus of this chapter.

Completing the picture

The glycaemic load of a food takes into account the glycaemic index of a specific food as well as the amount of carbs in a serving of that food. In summary, the glycaemic index is a *qualitative measure* and the glycaemic load is a *quantitative* one.

As explained, what the GI value of a food does not consider is the average portion size you eat at a meal or snack or how many carbohydrates there are in an average portion. For example, jam and carrots have similar GI ratings but you would have to eat platefuls of raw carrots – around 800g – for them to have a noticeable effect on your blood sugar, while just a dessertspoonful of jam would give you an instant sugar peak.

Because both the amount and type of carbohydrate are needed to predict blood glucose responses to a meal, we need a way to combine and define the two. Professor Walter Willett, Chairman of the Department of Nutrition at Harvard Medical School, did this by coming up with the term 'glycaemic load'. The glycaemic load is based around the GI but also factors in the carbohydrate content of a typical portion – or the amount of each food you would eat at one meal or snack. What it does is simplify the science behind the GI so you can use it in everyday life. It also corrects some of the inconsistencies on the glycaemic index that would technically limit foods that are perfectly good for you in reasonable amounts.

The good news about the GL is that it evens the playing field. A lot of foods that have a high GI rating actually have a low GL, for example carrots, sweetcorn and watermelon. So if you use the GL as your guide to healthy eating you actually have more food choices. You can choose foods from all the major food groups and enjoy a varied, satisfying and nutritious diet for the rest of your life. And the only side effect is weight loss and better health. Small wonder the GL has been described[10] as the most important breakthrough in diet and nutrition in the last fifty or so years.

How the GL is worked out

The GL gives values according to the effect on blood sugar of a normal portion of the food in question. For example, three or four slices of bread contain approximately 50g of carbohydrates, but to get 50g of carbohydrates from carrots you would need to eat 700g or 1½lb of carrots. A typical portion size for carrots is around 80–100g. The question is, what is the glycaemic response of a typical 90g portion size? If you don't want to do the maths, you can find a list of low GL foods online at: <www.mendosa.com> but for those who are interested, here's how to calculate the GL.

Take the GI rating and use the following equation:

Glycaemic load = GI rating divided by 100 times the number of grams of carbohydrate per serving

For instance, the GI rating of carrots is 75 so you would divide that number by 100: 75 divided by 100 = 0.75g. Then you would multiply that number by the carbohydrates in the portion. A 10g portion of carrots would contain around 7g of carbs: 0.75g x 7 = a GL of 5.25.

So although carrots have a high GI rating of 75, when the portion size is taken into account this becomes a low GL rating. This means you can eat your portion of carrots without worrying that they will interfere with your blood sugar balance and make you store fat. On the other hand, if you had just used the GI rating as a guide you'd have probably avoided carrots with their high rating of 75, thinking they would make you put on weight. Quite the opposite: carrots are not only extremely nutritious but when portion size is taken into account they have a very low glycaemic load, and it's the load that is important.

The same applies for many other foods that have a high GI rating but a low GL rating when average portion size is taken into account. Sugar, for instance is a very high GI food with a score of 100, but if only a teaspoon is eaten it will be a low GL with a score of 4.9. This isn't just a more accurate way of assessing the glycaemic impact of food in your diet, it is also far less restrictive and encourages you to eat a more varied and interesting diet.

Glycaemic load values are much lower than glycaemic index ones:

High GL = 20 or more
Medium GL = 11–19
Low GL = 10 or less

If one portion contains 12g of carbohydrate and the food item has a GI of 40 then the glycaemic load of the food is: (12 times 40) divided by 100 = 4.8 (rounded to 5). This food has both a low GI and a low GL.

If one portion contains 56g of carbohydrate and the food item has a GI of 45 then the glycaemic load of the food is: (56 times 45) divided by 100 = 25.2 (rounded to 25). Although this food item has a low GI of 45, the GL is high at 25, an indication that you should be careful with portion size and how frequently you eat this food item.

And here are a few more examples:

Spaghetti has a GI value of 40. A serving (1 cup) contains 52g of carbohydrate. The glycaemic load of spaghetti is: (40 times 52) divided by 100 = 20.8, which is high.

An apple has a GI value of 40. A serving (medium-sized apple) contains 15g of carbohydrate. The glycaemic load of an apple is: (40 times 15) divided by 100 = 6, which is low.

A potato has a GI value of 90 and 20g of carbohydrate per serving. It has a glycaemic load of (90 times 20) divided by 100 = 18, which is moderate.

It's also worth pointing out that the GI can mislead when it comes to certain foods that have a low GI rating. Take pasta, for example, which has a GI of less than 55 and is classed as low GI. With the GL an average portion size of around 180g has a GL rating of approximately 19 or 20, which means it is moderate to high GL.

Table 1 GI and GL for common foods

Food	GI	Serving size	Net carbs	GL
Peanuts	14	4oz (113g)	15	2
Bean sprouts	25	1 cup (104g)	4	1
Grapefruit	25	$\frac{1}{2}$ large (166g)	11	3
Pizza	30	2 slices (260g)	42	13
Low fat yogurt	33	1 cup (245g)	47	16
Apples	38	1 medium (138g)	16	6
Spaghetti	42	1 cup (140g)	38	16
Carrots	47	1 large (72g)	5	2
Oranges	48	1 medium (131g)	12	6
Bananas	52	1 large (136g)	27	14
Potato crisps	54	4oz (114g)	55	30
Snickers Bar	55	1 bar (113g)	64	35
Brown rice	55	1 cup (195g)	42	23
Honey	55	1 tbsp (21g)	17	9
Porridge	58	1 cup (234g)	21	12
Ice cream	61	1 cup (72g)	16	10
Macaroni and cheese	64	1 serving (166g)	47	30
Raisins	64	1 small box (43g)	32	20
White rice	64	1 cup (186g)	52	33
Sugar (sucrose)	68	1 tbsp (12g)	12	8
White bread	70	1 slice (30g)	14	10
Watermelon	72	1 cup (154g)	11	8
Popcorn	72	2 cups (16g)	10	7
Baked potato	85	1 medium (173g)	33	28
Glucose	100	(50g)	50	50

Table 1 shows values of the glycaemic index (GI) and glycaemic load (GL) for a few common foods. Remember, GIs of 55 or below are considered low, and those of 70 or above are considered high. GLs of 10 or below are considered low, and those of 20 or above are considered high.

As the table reveals, even foods with a high GI can have a low GL when the portion size is considered.

New evidence[11] associates high GL meals with an increased risk for heart disease and diabetes, especially in overweight and insulin-resistant people. Therefore, it is advisable to restrict the GL of a typical meal to between 20 and 25 as far as possible, but definitely to keep it below 30. The GL of a typical snack should preferably be between 10 and 15, but if your meals are all close to 30, the total of your snacks should be no more than 10. This means that you would have to eat fruit for snacks, in order to keep your total daily GL below 100, as the GL of fruit is usually below 10.

Don't worry about remembering the equation or doing calculations to determine your daily glycaemic load: there are plenty of low GI food lists to refer to and this book will help you assess what an average size portion is. The key thing to understand at this stage is that if you are eating a food with a high GI rating you can limit the effect it will have on your blood sugar and your weight by keeping the portion size small.

The glycaemic factor

Linking up the GI with the GL, which in this book is referred to as the *glycaemic factor*, gives a more complete picture and is by far a more accurate reference for healthy eating than the GI alone. It's a simple and effective way to make healthy food choices, and, as we'll see in the next chapter, lose weight at the same time.

Points to remember

- There is no such thing as a good or bad carbohydrate food. All carbohydrate foods can fit into a healthy diet – it all depends on when you eat it, how much you eat and with what you combine it.
- Rather than select foods solely based on their GI or GL, it's important to use your common sense and evaluate foods for their nutrition and health value.

- Foods with a high GI but low GL can be included as part of a healthy diet.
- When you eat foods with a high GI, the smaller the serving size, the smaller the rise in your blood sugar and insulin response.
- If low GI foods have a high GL they can affect blood glucose levels quite significantly if they are eaten in large amounts, especially if they are concentrated sources of carbohydrates, e.g. most cakes, dried fruit and dried fruit bars, fruit juices, crisps, chocolates, etc.
- High GI and high GL means trouble – blood glucose levels will shoot up. In general, low GL foods are whole, less processed foods including fresh fruits and vegetables, wholegrain breads, cereal and brown rice.
- The aim is to keep your total GL per day under 100.

4

The glycaemic factor and weight loss

If you want to lose weight, you need to stabilize your blood sugar levels. Study[12] after study has confirmed that this is by far the most important factor when it comes to burning away that excess body fat and keeping it off! The glycaemic factor diet focuses on helping you choose foods that will keep your blood sugar levels stable, and that's why it is such a successful weight loss tool.

The theory is that foods with a low glycaemic factor slowly release sugar into your blood, providing you with a steady, even supply of energy that leaves you feeling satisfied for longer. By contrast, foods with a high glycaemic factor cause a rapid – but short-lived – rise in blood sugar. The rapid rise in blood sugar triggers the production of insulin and, as we saw in the last few chapters, the storage of excess sugar as fat, which causes weight gain. Also, once blood sugar levels fall you'll be left feeling hungry and lacking in energy within a short time after eating, with the result that you end up reaching for a sugary, fatty snack to give you a boost and the whole cycle starts again. If this pattern is frequently repeated you'll be experiencing a roller-coaster of sugar highs and lows and overproduction of insulin, the hormone that causes your body to store fat.

In a nutshell, if you want to beat food cravings and lose weight, stabilizing your blood sugar levels and keeping your insulin levels low is absolutely crucial.

The glycaemic diet

Before the GI diet, most diets were based on the idea that if you restrict your intake of a particular type of food group – carbohydrates, proteins or fat – while satisfying your appetite with less fattening alternatives, you'll lose weight. Research[13] has now shown that restricting a particular food group can have a disastrous effect on a person's health and wellbeing. Scientists and doctors[14] generally approve of glycaemic diets for weight loss because they are not crash diets and they don't exclude important food groups. Instead they suggest a healthy, nutritious eating plan that can easily be followed for life.

There are now several detailed glycaemic diet plans available in book form that can help you get started, and a few of the most well known are outlined in brief below. You may want to follow one of these until you feel confident enough to go it alone. Alternatively you could just use the information in this book until you have enough understanding of how it works and can devise your own healthy weight loss plan.

Popular GI diets

The Jennie Brand-Miller Low GI Diet

Jennie Brand-Miller, PhD, is Professor of Human Nutrition at the University of Sydney. She has been spearheading GI research for the past three decades and is an acknowledged and respected expert in her field, with several books on the subject to her credit (see Further reading). After explaining the insulin response in detail, Brand-Miller outlines a 12-week low GI programme. Your gender, weight and activity levels are taken into consideration and matched up to an allotted number of servings per day. Every week of the plan you are given diet and exercise goals, with meal and exercise plans.

The diet urges you to eat plenty of vegetables, sweet potatoes, fruits, granary bread, stoneground bread, bulgar wheat, oats, basmati rice, beans, soya beans, nuts, nut butter, oily fish and plain yogurt. Foods to avoid or eat only occasionally include sweets, biscuits, crisps, cornflakes, corn pasta, canned spaghetti and short grain rice. You are also strongly advised to avoid large portions of any food.

If weight loss is your goal Brand-Miller typically advises:

- eating seven or more servings of fruit and vegetables a day;
- eating low GI breads and cereals;
- eating more beans, nuts, fish and seafood;
- eating low fat dairy products and lean red meat, poultry and eggs.

If weight maintenance is your goal she typically advises:

- don't skip meals;
- eat a good breakfast;
- eat four or five times a day;
- chose low GI carbs at every meal;
- eat lean protein at every meal;

33

- eat healthy fats i.e. omega 3 and 6;
- eat seven servings of fruit and vegetables a day;
- exercise for 30 to 60 minutes a day with one day off a week for relaxation.

Typical menu choices on a Brand-Miller GI diet
Breakfast:

- wholegrain toast with avocado and tomato;
- All-Bran with sliced banana and low fat milk;
- sourdough French toast with peaches;
- wholegrain toast with poached egg and grilled tomato;
- wholegrain toast with baked beans;
- wholegrain fruit loaf with ricotta.

Morning snack:

- fruit;
- dried fruit and nuts;
- roasted chickpeas;
- granola bar.

Lunch:

- pitta bread with hummus, salad and falafel;
- Greek salad with low fat feta and olives;
- chickpea and beetroot salad;
- thick vegetable soup;
- tuna and bean salad with garlic pitta toasts;
- wholegrain chicken, avocado and tomato toasted sandwich.

Afternoon snack:

- stoned wheat thins with avocado and tomato;
- pear and chocolate muffins;
- berries and low fat yogurt;
- raw nuts;
- low fat fruit smoothie.

Dinner:

- tomato and salmon pasta with salad;
- bean and corn burritos;
- fish and white bean salsa and salad;
- tandoori chicken with basmati rice;
- pasta with meat and roasted vegetables;
- pitta bread pizzas.

Dessert:

- fresh fruit;
- tinned fruit and custard;
- apple and rhubarb crumble;
- fruit salad with yogurt;
- poached pears in cranberry juice.

Brand-Miller's books are detailed, comprehensive and packed with lists and guidelines. The downside is that the plan is quite strict and does require quite a lot of preparation and planning, which may not suit everyone. The eating guidelines are, however, nutritious and healthy and if you decide to follow the diet you will certainly notice an improvement in your health and your weight.

The Rick Gallop GI Diet

Former president of the Heart and Stroke Foundation of Ontario, Canada, Rick Gallop began to investigate GI diets when a back injury stopped him exercising and he gained 20lb. Other diets didn't help him lose weight so he decided to devise his own, based on low GI foods. He spent many years experimenting with the diet to make it as simple and as easy to follow as possible. His books rate high GI foods in red, medium GI in yellow and low GI in green.

Before starting the programme Gallop urges you to choose a target weight based on a body mass index (BMI   see p. 41) of between 22 and 25. He recommends a visualization exercise where you imagine the amount of weight you want to lose and then see yourself carrying it around in bags of sugar in a backpack all day. The feeling of relief when you take the backpack off should help motivate you to start his diet programme.

Gallop's diet has two phases. In phase 1 you are urged to remove all red and amber foods from your cupboard and to shop only for green foods, which are all low calorie, low fat and high fibre. You also need to record your weight and to weigh yourself on a daily basis. During phase 1 portions of meat and fish should weigh no more than 100g, dry pasta should weigh no more than 40g and rice no more than 50g. You are urged to eat three meals and three snacks a day. During phase 1 you are only to eat foods from the green list until you reach your target weight. Once you reach your target weight you enter phase 2 and can now begin to add amber GI foods and increase your calorie intake; but plenty of exercise is advised, as is regular weighing to make sure the weight doesn't creep back on.

Gallop's GI diet rules include:

- Eat three meals and three snacks a day.
- Restrict portion sizes of meat, pasta and rice.
- Keep the ratio of carbohydrates, protein and fat.
- Eat plenty of fruits and vegetables.
- Drink plenty of water.
- Exercise for 30 minutes a day.

Green light foods to enjoy during phase 1 include: oats and high fibre cereals, fruits and fruit juice but not bananas and dates, salads, most vegetables, lean skinless chicken and turkey, oily fish, nuts, cottage cheese, basmati rice, omega 3 eggs, skimmed milk, All-Bran, beans, low fat cottage cheese, stoneground wholemeal bread, almonds, hazelnuts.

Foods that can be reintroduced during phase 2 include: bananas, sweetcorn cobs, low fat ice cream, pasta, boiled potatoes, wine and caffeinated drinks.

Foods to avoid during phase 1 include: butter, bacon, whole eggs, chips, baguettes, alcohol, caffeinated drinks and any desserts.

Foods to avoid or eat sparingly during phase 2 include: large portions of any food, fried or mashed potato, beer, chocolate, sugar-coated breakfast cereals, biscuits, fish and meat in batter and breadcrumbs.

Sample menus

Breakfast choices:

- porridge;
- egg white omelette;
- bran cereal;
- fresh fruit;
- low fat cottage cheese.

Mid-morning and mid-afternoon snack choices:

- raw vegetables;
- fruit yogurt;
- fresh fruit.

Lunch choices:

- vegetable soup;
- vegetable salad;
- pasta salad.

Dinner choices:

- baked fish on a bed of leeks and onions;
- meat loaf.

Gallop's diet is clear and well planned. The red, amber and green listing of foods certainly makes for ease of reference and if you stick to his recommendations it's highly likely that you will lose weight, although the book doesn't address such issues as stress hormones and toxins. Gallop focuses on foods that are both low calorie and low GI and the recipes and meal plans are interesting. The only downside is that many medium and high GI foods are banned and this could lead to food cravings. The programme also doesn't address glycaemic load at all but instead gives you recommended serving sizes, so if you use this programme you need to be sure you don't eat too high a glycaemic load. It also recommends the use of artificial sweeteners and several studies have expressed concerns about their effects on health.

The GI Plan: Azmina Govindji and Nina Puddefoot

Govindji, a former dietician for Diabetes UK, and Puddefoot, a life development coach, base their GI plan on low GI foods but each food is given a point value known as a 'GiP'. For the first two weeks of the diet women are allowed 17 points a day and men 22. In the third week points rise to 20 for women and 25 for men and stay that way until target weight is reached. Once target weight has been reached points rise to 23 for women and 28 for men. You are advised to eat three meals a day and three snacks and to lose no more than 1kg a week. The book is also packed with meal plans, recipes, motivational tips, lifestyle advice and affirmations.

Foods to enjoy on the GI plan include fresh fruit, fresh vegetables, bran and oat cereals, granary and wholemeal bread, brown and basmati rice, beans and lentils, olive oil, pasta, low fat yogurt, fish, quorn and plenty of water. Foods to avoid include white bread, sweet fizzy drinks, chips, mashed potato, fatty meat, pastries, cakes, meat pies, biscuits, rice cakes, jasmine rice and confectionery.

A typical daily menu might be:

- breakfast – granary bread and scrambled egg;
- lunch – jacket potato with tuna and sweetcorn;
- dinner – salmon steak in garlic balsamic dressing with fettucine and steamed asparagus tips, followed by fresh fruit;
- snacks – almonds, packet of soup.

If you stick to the points system in the book there's every chance you'll lose weight without going hungry and without missing out on nutrients. Eating out could be a problem as the book tends to focus on only the plainest of foods. The daily motivational tips may not suit everyone's taste and you may also find the points system restrictive and difficult to fit into real life.

Antony Worrall Thompson's GI Diet

Celebrity chef Antony Worrall Thompson created this diet to help prevent diabetes after he was diagnosed with syndrome X (see p. 53). He is keen to stress the importance of enjoying food and explains that you won't feel hungry on his diet as low GI foods take longer to digest than those with a higher GI. The book is packed with cooking guidelines, advice on nutrition and delicious recipes.

Foods to enjoy on the GI diet include stir fries with beans and vegetables, basmati rice, fruit, fruit crumbles made with oats, poached egg, lean bacon, baked fish, lentil soup, new potatoes cooked in their skins, pitta bread with salad and baked beans on toast.

Foods to avoid include biscuits, white rice, liver, egg yolks, shellfish, sweet drinks, creamy sauces, fish in batter and pastries.

Sample daily menu:

- breakfast – porridge with berry fruits;
- lunch – roast chicken with sweet potatoes;
- dinner – barley and goat's cheese soufflé;
- snacks – pancakes and honey, soda bread roll.

This diet is effective as long as you have the discipline to be strict about your portion sizes. The recipes are delicious and as it's not a complicated or difficult diet to follow it will suit those who enjoy a more relaxed approach to nutrition.

The GL Diet: Nigel Denby

Nigel Denby is a qualified chef and dietician with his own private practice in Harley Street. His GL or glycaemic load diet focuses attention on the glycaemic load rather than low GI food ratings. The book stresses the importance of eating three meals a day and snacks in between to keep blood sugar levels stable, as well as regular exercise, avoiding trigger foods and monitoring portion size. There are no phases and stages to the diet. Instead the reader is urged to plunge straight in with the GL diet plan which is billed as a permanent life change. There is also a helpful guide to eating out and plenty of basic, simple recipes with ingredients that are easy to buy in a supermarket.

Foods to enjoy on Denby's GL diet include salads with lemon or vinegar, fresh fruit and vegetables, oat bran, couscous, sweet potatoes, yams, swede, pumpernickel bread, unprocessed lean cuts of meat and fish, free range eggs, nuts and low fat dairy products. Foods to eat sparingly if you're trying to lose weight include full fat dairy products, fatty meats, sugar, sugary snacks, white bread, pasta and rice, dried fruit, corn products, chips, mashed potatoes and baked potatoes.

Sample daily menu:

- breakfast – reduced-sugar baked beans on toasted low GL bread;
- lunch – poached fish with salad and dressing;
- dinner – cottage cheese salad with olive oil dressing;
- snacks – soup, watermelon, cheese sticks and fruit.

The GL diet is nutritionally sound, and if you can get your head around the concept of the glycaemic load and follow the eating plan you should be able to lose weight without feeling hungry. There are no complicated GL calculations to do as the book lists them all for you. There is also no dictatorial regime to adhere to so you can fit this diet around your lifestyle, rather than building your life around the diet.

Easy GI Diet: Helen Foster

Helen Foster is a health writer and her accessible book outlines how a low GI diet can give you more energy and protect against heart disease and diabetes, as well as assisting weight loss. It clearly explains what the glycaemic index is, and exactly how it can help you to lose weight. Foods with a low GI index – which convert to glucose slowly, keeping hunger at bay for longer – are detailed. You can choose from one of four diet plans, which feature a variety of recipes: 14-day GI genius plan; 14-day GI vegetarian plan; GI galvanizer plan; GI for life plan.

The book splits recipes for meat eaters and vegetarians into sections. Each of the sections includes two weeks' worth of menus including breakfast, lunch, dinner and snacks. Most of the recipes take about ten minutes to prepare and are ideal for people with busy lives. The whole family can eat, and benefit from, the food prepared, as it is a balanced, sensible diet. There are suggestions for how to exercise, and how to fit regular exercise into your daily routine. For people looking for an easy-to-follow guide the *Easy GI Diet* ticks all the boxes.

In addition to the above, Barry Sear's Zone Diet and Ann Louise Gittleman's Fat Flush Plan are also good weight loss programmes that can assist you in eating based on the glycaemic index. It's impossible, however, to list all the variations and varieties of mainstream GI diet guides, cookbooks and recipes for weight loss here, but hopefully the above has given you a taster of what is mainstream and readily available. If you don't want to invest in another book the guidelines below can help you make all the long-term changes you need to achieve your desired weight and get all the nutrients you need for good health from a well-balanced diet.

Glycaemic factor weight loss guidelines

It's a good idea before beginning any weight loss programme to decide what would be a healthy weight for you to reach. It's pointless to set unrealistic goals. If you have a naturally curvy body, trying to lose too much weight will just make you look and feel weak and ill. If you're a tall person with a large frame, setting your goal to be a size 6 is unrealistic but perhaps a 14, 12 or even a 10 is within the range of possibility. If you exercise a lot you'll have more muscle, which will make you look slimmer and fitter, but because muscle weighs more than fat you may weigh more than someone who is less active.

Each one of us has a natural weight range and you need to find out what your natural weight range is. Height and weight charts give an idea of that range but by no means an accurate one. Two people of the same height and build can have very different ideal weights and still be healthy. Because of this doctors tend to refer to the body mass index or BMI to see if a person is overweight or not. The BMI is a height to weight formula that gives an indication of total body fat.

To calculate your BMI divide your weight in kilograms by the square of your height in metres. For example, you might be 1.6m (5 feet 3 inches) tall and weigh 65kg (10 stone). The calculation would then be:

1.6 x 1.6 = 2.56. BMI would be 65 divided by 2.56 = 25.39

If you don't want to do the maths there are plenty of BMI calculators on the internet (e.g. www.bbc.co.uk/health/healthy_living/ your_weight/bmiimperial_index.shtml, nhlbisupport.com/bmi/ or www.cdc.gov/nccdphp/dnpa/bmi/calc-bmi.htm) that can calculate it for you. Once you've found out your BMI, check the following to see if you fall into the average range:

• below 15: severely underweight;
• 15–19: underweight;
• 19–25: average;
• 25–30: overweight;
• 30–40: obese (if this is you, consult your doctor for weight loss advice as you could be endangering your health).

Another measure that doctors use is the waist to hip ratio. Waist measurements of more than 102cm (40 inches) for men and more than 89cm (35 inches) for women have been linked with all sorts of health problems, in particular heart disease. To find out your waist to hip ratio, divide your waist measurement by your hip measurement. Above 1.0 for men and 0.85 for women increases your risk of heart disease.

Your ideal weight is the weight where you feel healthy, comfortable and energetic. How much weight do you have to lose to take you down into your average BMI range? This is the weight you should be aiming for.

Aim for slow and steady weight loss

Once you have determined what weight you are going to aim for, set a weekly or monthly weight loss goal. Aim for slow and steady here. If you lose it quickly you are likely to put it all back on just as quickly as soon as you eat 'normally' again. If you want to lose 10kg, you need to give yourself at least three or four months, and if you want to lose more than that you need to allow six months to a year. Ideally you should lose no more than 1kg a week and a realistic target is to lose 5 to 10 per cent of your starting body weight within six months.

You will start to feel better after a few days on a glycaemic factor diet but don't expect the weight to drop off immediately. Take things slowly, one day at a time, and aim for a gradual rather than a fast weight loss as research[15] has shown that slow and gradual weight loss is the most effective way to lose weight and keep it off. If this seems discouraging, just know that weight loss takes as long as it takes but the end result – your ideal shape – is to keep.

Note: if you want to lose weight you should consult your doctor if you have a medical condition, are on any medication or are pregnant or planning to be. You should also speak to your doctor if you have more than 5kg to lose or are planning to start an exercise programme and haven't exercised for a long time.

The glycaemic factor weight loss diet is a balanced diet

Once you've got a realistic weight loss goal in mind, and have consulted your doctor, you can begin a glycaemic factor weight loss diet according to the glycaemic factor diet guidelines given in this book.

The low glycaemic load approach to weight management differs significantly from low carbohydrate and low fat diets because eating foods with a low glycaemic rating encourages those on a weight loss programme to eat nutritious foods from all food groups. To lose and manage weight you use the GI and GL as tools to help you choose from a wide variety of healthy carbohydrates. Combine these with lean protein and heart-healthy essential fats for a nutritious well-balanced diet.

Try not to forget that eating low GI and GL carbohydrates isn't the whole story. To burn fat effectively you need nutrients from all the food groups, and it's also very important that you eat low fat protein sources and healthy fats, like fish oils, nuts and seeds, as both have a stabilizing effect on blood sugar. You should also drink lots of water and eat plenty of fresh fruits, vegetables, legumes, whole grains and pulses. Foods to avoid include heavily processed and refined foods with additives, preservatives, sugar and salt and foods high in saturated fat such as animal and dairy products.

Your daily glycaemic load allotment

The key to weight loss with the glycaemic factor is really very simple: eat within your glycaemic load allotment every day. Here are some guidelines for choosing that allotment. Start with these and then lower them if you are not losing weight or raise them if you are losing weight too quickly. Start with a glycaemic load allotment of between 60 and 75 per day. (Increase this to between 100 or 150 if you need to be very active.) Eat three meals and three snacks a day with, say, 15 at each meal and 10 at each snack.

If you don't want to calculate your glycaemic load you can still count carbohydrates. To start allow yourself 30g of low glycaemic carbohydrates per meal and 10–30 low glycaemic carbohydrates for snacks. The carbohydrate total for the day should be less than 150; most people lose weight with a carbohydrate total between 90 and 120.

After three or four weeks you'll soon get an idea of how the carbohydrates are working in your body. If you aren't losing weight, lower your glycaemic load allotment to 50 or 60 until you do start to lose weight. It's not recommended for anyone to go lower than a 50 glycaemic load.

Get snacking

It's really important on a glycaemic factor weight loss programme to eat three meals a day and at least three snacks. Start with a good breakfast, have a mid-morning snack, followed by lunch, a mid-afternoon snack and then supper and a snack before bedtime.

Lots of people trying to lose weight make the mistake of skipping breakfast, having a light lunch and then eating a large evening meal. Stacking your calories up like this isn't a good idea because in the fasting state your body does the best that it can to cling on to every last calorie, effectively reducing your metabolic rate. Then when you do eventually eat in the evening your body is set to store as much fat as possible. Also after eating you often go to bed so your body has little time to use up the calories you have just consumed.

Missing breakfast and going for long periods without eating triggers your body's fat storage system with a rapid increase in blood sugar levels and insulin. Starting the day with breakfast kick starts your metabolism so it is in fat-burning mode all day long. Regular meals and snacks throughout the day ensure that your blood sugars remain stable, you aren't feeling hungry all the time and weight loss is encouraged.

Portion control

Every meal you eat should be a nutritious balance of carbohydrates, proteins and healthy fats. If you follow the glycaemic diet guidelines in Chapters 2 and 3 you should be getting a balanced diet. Just watch your portion size. As a rough guide, here is a GI friendly food pyramid:

- Two servings of meat, fish, poultry, eggs a day. Red meat no more than twice a week. One serving = one egg, or meat and fish about the size of a clenched fist.
- One to three servings of nuts, seeds and legumes a day and oils made from these. One serving = half a cup of beans, a handful of nuts and seeds.
- Two to three servings of low fat milk, yogurt and cheese a day (or of non-dairy produce such as soya or nut milk). One serving = about 2oz of cheese or 1 cup of milk or yogurt.
- Three to six servings of starchy carbohydrates (granary bread, grains, pasta, rice, cereals) a day. One serving = one slice of bread, one bowl of cereal or half a cup of rice or pasta.
- Two to three servings of fruit a day. One serving = one piece of fruit.
- Five servings of vegetables a day. One serving = half a cup of raw or cooked vegetables.
- Fats and oils should be eaten in moderation. White bread, rice, potatoes and sugary treats should be eaten only rarely.

Portion sizes have got bigger and bigger over the years and waistlines have followed suit. Proper attention to serving size will encourage the slow, gradual weight loss you should aim for. Go for average and not supersize portions at each meal. A good guide is not to eat at one sitting more than you could fit into your cupped hands. Another guide is to look at your plate: about half of it should be filled with vegetables, a quarter with starchy carbohydrates and a quarter with protein.

If you are concerned that smaller portions won't satisfy your hunger, remember that regular meals and snacks throughout the day will help curb your appetite. It's also a good idea to take your time over your meals. Put your knife and fork down after each mouthful and chew your food thoroughly. It takes around 10 or 15 minutes for your stomach to send messages to your brain that you are full, so if you think you want to eat more try waiting 15 minutes to see if you are really hungry or just overeating.

There are, of course, some foods that you don't need to be so strict about when it comes to portion size. You can eat as much as you like of foods, such as vegetables, that are both low GI and low GL, and you'll find plenty of those listed in Chapter 8.

Exercise

Exercise, in combination with a glycaemic factor diet, is an essential tool for anyone who wants to lose weight and maintain their weight loss. Most weight loss experts stress the importance of increasing your activity levels on a weight loss programme.

Calorie counting isn't typically stressed on a glycaemic diet, but whether you count calories or not the weight gain equation remains the same: if you eat more calories than you burn off you'll gain weight. Exercise is a great way to burn off calories. For example, if you want to lose weight you need to reduce your calorie intake by around 500 calories a day. Half an hour of jogging can burn off 200 calories, 30 minutes of brisk walking could burn off 150 calories. This means if you are exercising you won't need to cut back so much on what you eat.

But the benefits of exercise don't stop there. Exercise also speeds up your metabolism and the effects last way beyond your workout. Studies show that fit people burn more calories even when they are resting, because it takes more calories to maintain muscle tissue than fat tissue. Once you increase the muscle in your body you will be burning more calories even when you are doing something sedentary like sitting reading this book! So the more you exercise, the more your muscles build up and the speedier your metabolism becomes.

There's another reason why exercise is so important for weight loss. Recent research confirms that regular, moderate exercise lowers blood sugar levels and promotes insulin efficiency, which as we've seen is the key to weight loss. Exercise also stimulates the release of endorphins which relieve stress and make you feel good about yourself. Making exercise a regular part of your life is a great way to boost weight loss and boost self-esteem at the same time. So if you're serious about losing weight try setting aside a minimum of 30 minutes a day for walking, biking, dancing, jogging, football, netball, tennis, an exercise class or video or whatever activity you enjoy the most. If you can't set aside 30 minutes in one go, try exercising for three lots of ten minutes – it can be just as beneficial.

Drink plenty of water a day

Water is essential to life. The nutrients we get from food are transported around the body by water and most of the chemical reactions in the body need water. Water is vital for hormone function and research has shown that metabolic rate increases after drinking water. Water also keeps you from mistaking thirst for hunger. Most of us simply don't get enough water. You should aim for 1.5 to 2 litres a day; that's around eight to nine glasses. You'll know if you are dehydrated if your urine is dark and not pale or straw coloured as it should be.

The 80–20 rule

As far as possible go for healthy, fresh food and avoid food that has been processed and refined. Processed and refined foods are likely to be high in sugar and salt and additives. Additives add to the body's toxic load, salt increases the risk of high blood pressure and sugar interferes with insulin function. Caffeine and alcohol should also be avoided as they are stimulants which can upset blood sugar balance.

But what if you slip and can't resist the odd bar of chocolate, can of pepsi or beer or bag of chips? If this happens and you find yourself munching on foods that you know are going to set your blood sugar levels soaring such as doughnuts first thing in the morning or pigging out at dinner last night, don't beat yourself up about it. It's impossible to eat healthily all the time and the occasional indulgence – bar of chocolate or packet of crisps – doesn't mean you have failed. It is the excesses that are dangerous. If you make sure you follow the glycaemic factor diet guidelines 80 per cent of the time you can allow yourself the occasional indulgence and still lose weight.

Rest and relaxation

You may find it hard to believe but regular relaxation can help you lose weight.

This is because when you're stressed the adrenal glands prompt the release of sugar stores into your bloodstream. If you are under long-term stress and no way is found to release or deal with that stress, sugar stays too long in your system and your body is driven towards insulin imbalance and weight gain.

Deal with minor stress (such as missing a train or sitting in a traffic jam) with simple relaxation techniques such as tensing your muscles hard and then relaxing them. Other techniques for short-term stress include stretching regularly, deep breathing, soaking in a warm bath, getting a good night's sleep, drinking herbal teas like chamomile, having a good laugh, stroking a pet or simply day dreaming. If stress is more serious, such as the threat of redundancy or the end of a relationship, it's important that you set aside time to relax every day no matter what. Meditation, massage and yoga are great ways to unwind. Exercise can also reduce stress and boost energy, but perhaps one of the best ways to ease stress is to talk to friends, family and partners. If you don't feel you have anyone to talk to a trained counsellor may help you get in touch with your feelings and give you tips on how to deal with stress.

Not getting a good night's sleep can also contribute towards weight gain. Research findings[16] show that, in addition to raising stress hormones, sleep deprivation disrupts hormonal balance, interferes with blood sugar levels, makes you feel anxious, causes you to age prematurely and increases the risk of weight gain and poor health. A good night's sleep is the best tonic you can have, but it's important to realize that quality and not quantity is the key. A recent study[17] showed that a good night's sleep makes people happier, but those who had less than six hours' or over ten hours' sleep became irritable. Seven or eight hours seems ample for most people, but six hours of good-quality sleep beats a restless ten.

A little extra help

It seems that adding vinegar to your meals can prove helpful. Experts aren't entirely sure why but studies[18] show that acetic acid, the chief acid of vinegar, seems to be able to lower blood glucose levels. In one study the glucose response with vinegar was 31 per cent lower than without it. If you don't like vinegar try something else acidic, such as lemon or lime juice. Your best bet is to include a side salad with an olive oil and vinegar or lemon dressing in as many meals as possible.

Weight loss supplements

People with weight to lose can sometimes be deficient in major nutrients, especially those that increase metabolism and burn fat. A healthy, balanced diet should offset these deficiencies but here are some supplements you might want to consider taking:

- vitamin B complex: essential for efficient metabolism of carbohy-drates and proteins;

- co-enzyme Q10: helps stimulate the metabolism and weight loss;
- vitamin C: can help speed up a slow metabolism;
- boron: a US Department of Agriculture study revealed that this trace mineral may speed the burning of calories;
- amino acids L-ornithine, l-arginine and L-lysine: research has shown that weight loss can be improved with the use of combination of these amino acids;
- psyllium husks: for fibre to help cleanse your system and promote a feeling of fullness;
- digestive enzyme supplements: help boost nutrient uptake and suppress appetite;
- hemp seed oil: provides exactly the right combination of essential fatty acids to control appetite, boost metabolism and weight loss;
- kelp: helps support the thyroid gland and aid weight loss;
- lecithin: helps utilize body fat;
- chickweed: helps break down fat deposits that are hard to shift;
- nettle tea: a great weight loss tea as it boosts metabolism and is a natural appetite suppressant;
- spirulina: rich in protein, this can help control blood sugar swings and food cravings;
- kombucha tea has also shown promising results and helps to boost energy.

Also helpful would be a good multivitamin and mineral complex with potassium, calcium and zinc, which are all important for the production of energy.

Note: always consult with your GP or a nutritionist before taking supplements. You also need to remember that they won't help a great deal unless you combine your supplement programme with healthy diet and exercise.

Not a diet but a way of life

Perhaps the most important thing to remember when you begin a glycaemic factor diet is that permanent weight loss isn't actually about dieting. The word 'diet' in this book isn't used to refer to an attempt to lose weight by eating or cutting calories: it is used to describe the food you eat in general as well as specific foods that you should aim to eat on a regular basis. The glycaemic factor diet is about changing the way you eat for the rest of your life. It is about feeding your body the nutrients it needs to balance your blood sugar levels and keep insulin levels low so you can lose weight and maintain that weight loss in the long term.

If you follow the recommendations above, research[19] indicates that there is every chance that you can and will lose weight and, as you'll see in the next chapter, the only side effect is a healthier, happier you.

5

Health benefits of the glycaemic factor diet

The glycaemic factor diet is increasingly becoming popular as a weight loss tool but research[20] also indicates that it can benefit your health in numerous other ways. A glycaemic diet can affect a number of serious diseases, including obesity, syndrome X, diabetes, heart disease and cancer. It can also affect your mood and energy levels. Below you'll see how using a glycaemic diet can not only help reduce your risk of premature aging and certain diseases but also increases your chances of optimum physical, emotional and mental health and wellbeing.

Obesity

Despite all the diets currently available and the billions of people who are on a diet of some kind, the number of overweight and obese people in Western society is on the increase. It has been estimated that one in ten deaths in the UK and US may be related to or caused by obesity. This makes obesity second only to smoking as a preventable cause of death.

Around 64 per cent of American and British adults are currently believed to be overweight or obese. And with childhood obesity statistics reaching an unprecedented 30 per cent, some experts believe that within a few decades almost every adult will be struggling with their weight in some way. Excess weight carries with it a number of health concerns, from fatigue and aches and pains to serious health problems such as heart disease, diabetes and some types of cancer.

Although other problems, such as diabetes, stress, an underactive thyroid and hormonal disorders like PCOS, can contribute to obesity, the most common causes of obesity are overeating, lack of exercise and a poor diet. Many experts[21] today also attribute the rise in obesity to overconsumption of high glycaemic index foods, and the resulting overproduction of insulin which triggers weight gain. While it is more complex than many would admit, the evidence is growing to support a strong connection between high glycaemic foods and obesity. This is not the last word on this subject by any means, as research into the relationship between insulin levels and obesity is ongoing. However, the overconsumption of high GI foods is a major cause of concern.

If you are overweight the chances are you have already tried to lose weight by going on a weight-reducing diet. The trouble is, diets that reduce your calorie intake often end up making you fatter. This is because most diets urge you to reduce your carbohydrate and fat intake to lose weight quickly. The weight you lose, however, is mostly water which is stored with carbohydrates and muscles as muscle is broken down to produce glucose. Then when you return to your normal way of eating you put all the weight back on again and gain more fat. If this goes on for a number of years your body composition will have more fat and less muscle. Muscles are calorie burners and the less muscle you have the harder it can be to lose weight.

As concern about obesity grows, scientists are paying more attention to the role that the glycaemic load of foods plays in weight control. Clinical studies[22] have clearly shown that low glycaemic diets that stabilize blood sugar levels can help promote weight loss and decrease body fat, indicating that they have far greater potential for weight loss than low fat and low carbohydrate diets.

Diabetes and insulin resistance

An estimated 18 million American and 2 million Britons are diagnosed with diabetes every year. And, even more alarming, it's estimated that millions of people have the disease, or an increased risk of the disease, but don't know that they have it until they develop one of its life-threatening complications such as blindness, kidney disease, heart disease, stroke or nerve damage.

Diabetes isn't just hard to live with – it can be dangerous. It is currently one of the top ten causes of death in the US and the UK. Basically, people with diabetes have a problem with insulin. As we've seen, when insulin isn't doing its job, glucose can't get into your cells and accumulates in your blood, so that blood sugar levels get higher and higher.

Type 1 diabetes typically occurs in childhood and is thought to be genetic or caused by infections that damage the pancreas. Type 1 diabetics don't produce enough insulin and need to inject insulin to bring their blood sugar levels down.

Type 2 diabetes usually occurs later in life and is the most common form of diabetes. People with type 2 diabetes usually produce plenty of insulin but they have insulin resistance, which means their insulin doesn't work very well. People with type 2 diabetes can reduce their insulin resistance and bring their blood sugar glucose levels down with diet and lifestyle changes and sometimes with drugs as well.

Before full-blown type 2 diabetes sets in, there are various stages that bring a person closer to diabetes. Terms you might hear include prediabetes, hyperinsulinamea, impaired fasting glucose, impaired glucose tolerance and insulin resistance. All these terms refer to higher than normal amounts of insulin or glucose circulating in the blood. If nothing is done to lower these amounts, after several years the insulin-producing cells in the pancreas start to wear out and stop working. Insulin levels fall, blood sugar levels rise and rise and diabetes is diagnosed.

Research[23] indicates that high glycaemic diets increase insulin levels and the risk of diabetes, whereas low glycaemic diets reduce the risk. Unfortunately, you can't cure diabetes once it sets in, but diets containing low GI foods have been shown to improve blood sugar control in people with both type 1 and type 2 diabetes. It is possible, however, to reverse insulin resistance and reduce your risk of developing diabetes in the first place with a low glycaemic load diet. Diabetes prevention programmes[24] clearly demonstrate that low glycaemic load diets, when combined with regular exercise, can reverse prediabetic conditions and significantly reduce your risk of getting this chronic disease.

Heart disease

Heart disease is by far the biggest cause of death among American and British men and women. Nearly 62 million Americans have some form of cardiovascular disease, and nearly a million die from such conditions each year. In the UK, some 268,000 people have heart attacks each year, while 1.5 million men and 1.2 million women live with the disease.

So what causes this deadly disease? It is often caused by a condition known as atherosclerosis or hardening of the arteries. As people get older atherosclerosis tends to happen very gradually and most of us are unaware of it happening, but if its development is fast tracked by certain risk factors, the condition can become serious or even life-threatening.

Risk factors for heart disease include smoking, stress, physical inactivity, weight gain, high blood pressure, high cholesterol, high homocystein and high triglyceride levels. Knowing the risk factors means you can take action now to protect yourself, and studies[25] show that preventative measures are really effective in cutting your risk of heart disease. You can stop smoking, you can start exercising and you can combat high blood pressure and weight gain by switching to a low glycaemic diet.

A low glycaemic diet[26] helps fight heart disease by increasing your body's sensitivity to insulin so weight loss is easier. It improves your blood cholesterol levels by increasing good high density lipoprotein (HDL) cholesterol and reducing bad low density lipoprotein (LDL) cholesterol. It also lowers levels of homocystein, an amino acid, and triglycerides, a toxic form of fat. High cholesterol, homocystein and triglyceride levels have all been shown to increase the risk of heart disease.

Scientists[27] have now confirmed what has been suspected for a long time: a high glycaemic diet can increase the risk of cardiovascular disease and a low glycaemic diet can reduce risk. Studies[28] from the Harvard School of Public Health indicate that the risk of heart disease is strongly related to the GI of the overall diet. In 1999 the World Health Organization and Food and Agriculture Organization recommended that people in industrialized countries base their diets on low GI foods to prevent not just obesity and diabetes but heart disease too.

Syndrome X

Syndrome X is a term used to describe a set of factors found to significantly increase the risk of both heart disease and diabetes. These factors include elevated insulin levels (insulin resistance), central obesity (around the middle of the body – the classic 'apple' shape), high levels of blood fats – LDL (bad) cholesterol and triglycerides – and high blood pressure (hypertension).

The disorder is caused by your body's inability to make the most of the food you eat. Two of the key players in syndrome X are glucose and insulin. As we've seen already, the typical Western diet high in sugary foods and refined carbohydrates creates levels of glucose and insulin that are too high for our bodies to cope with. In the correct amounts glucose and insulin help our bodies metabolize food and burn energy and fat, but in high doses they confuse the metabolism and encourage the development of syndrome X.

In other words, syndrome X is caused primarily by a high glycaemic diet that not only raises glucose and insulin to unhealthy levels but also fails to supply the many nutrients the body needs to protect us from disease. The good news is that studies[29] suggest that the safest and most effective therapy to reduce the risk of syndrome X is a low glycaemic load diet along with regular exercise.

Cancer

According to a number of recent studies[30] a high dietary glycaemic load may increase the risk of colorectal (colon) cancer, breast cancer, ovarian cancer, gastric cancer, endometrial cancer and pancreatic cancer.

One of the major benefits of going on a glycaemic diet is that you will reduce your insulin levels. Although research on the connections between carbohydrates and cancer is still in its infancy at this stage, it does seem to provide confirming evidence that elevated insulin levels are a major factor that contributes to the growth of all cancers.

According to the research, only diets with high glycaemic loads – that is, diets rich in processed foods like white bread, white rice and other foods made from refined grains (cakes, biscuits, crisps, etc.) as well as other high glycaemic foods like potatoes and corn – are associated with an increased risk of cancer. The carbohydrates at the lower end of the glycaemic scale, such as vegetables and products made from whole grains, are not associated with increased risk. In fact, numerous studies[31] have shown for years that diets rich in a variety of vegetables, fruits, whole grains and legumes are consistently associated with lower cancer risk in general, and lower colorectal cancer risk in particular. So every time you substitute your sugary snack with a serving of vegetables you will take a huge proactive step towards preventing cancer.

Although research is still inconclusive some cancer experts believe that cancer patients can have a major improvement in their conditions if they control the supply of cancer's preferred fuel: glucose. While cancer cells derive most of their energy from glucose, the goal is not to eliminate sugars or carbohydrates entirely from the diet but rather to control blood glucose within a narrow range to help starve the cancer cells and boost immune function. By slowing the cancer's growth, patients make it possible for their immune systems to be strengthened.

In short, controlling blood glucose levels through a low glycaemic load diet combined with exercise, supplements and stress reduction could be one of the most crucial components to a cancer treatment and prevention programme.

Premenstrual syndrome (PMS)

Medical research suggests that up to 90 per cent of women experience symptoms of PMS, and that 40 per cent find that it interferes with their daily lives. PMS is a complex disorder with wide-ranging symptoms, causes and treatments. And while there are still plenty of unsolved mysteries surrounding this condition, medical experts[32] all agree on one thing: eating too much sugar makes PMS worse.

This is because during the week before a woman's period her body becomes extra-responsive to insulin. When insulin clears away the glucose, this can cause fatigue and cravings for sweets. Eating sugar stimulates the release of large amounts of insulin again, the same substance that caused blood sugar levels to plummet in the first place. It's a vicious cycle that can trigger many of the symptoms typically associated with PMS such as mood swings, fatigue and irritability.

Too much sugar also overworks the liver, making it less able to process the sex hormone oestrogen effectively. Oestrogen levels rise and a woman can feel bloated, irritable and anxious. Besides increasing oestrogen levels, too much sugar is also associated with a lowering of progesterone, which many experts believe to be a major trigger for symptoms of PMS. (Progesterone is the hormone that is vital for a successful pregnancy; and blood sugar imbalances have been associated with fertility problems.)

Watching your blood glucose levels and avoiding high sugar and sugary foods especially during the week or so before a period is strongly advised by doctors and nutritionists. A healthy PMS eating plan aims to stabilize blood sugar levels to help prevent the sugar cravings, as well as the mood swings and fatigue associated with PMS. And the best way to balance your blood sugar is to eat carbohydrates that have a low glycaemic value.

Polycystic ovary syndrome (PCOS)

PCOS is a metabolic disorder that affects as many as one in ten women. Symptoms include irregular or absent periods, weight gain, acne, oily skin and facial and body hair. It is the number one cause of infertility and, if left untreated, can increase the risk of endometrial cancer. In addition, women with PCOS are at a greater risk for heart disease and diabetes.

Until recently, diet was not thought of as an important adjunct in treatment. However, since the fairly recent discovery regarding the role of insulin resistance in PCOS many experts[33] now believe that diet should be a part of the treatment plan. Although further research is needed, it is believed that diet can help reduce insulin resistance in women with PCOS, which can not only help erratic periods, unwanted hair growth and acne, but may decrease the risk of heart disease and diabetes as well.

Exactly why and how PCOS develops is not quite clear; however, most experts[34] now agree that insulin plays a major role in triggering the release of higher levels of androgens (male hormones) which leads to irregular periods, acne and other typical PCOS symptoms. Although not all women with PCOS are insulin resistant, the majority are and the discovery of insulin's role in PCOS has improved treatment options. Treatment is no longer just aimed at treating the individual symptoms, such as irregular periods and acne, but instead is now aimed at treating one of the underlying causes – insulin resistance. If insulin resistance is present, it is best treated with a low glycaemic index diet, exercise and weight loss if needed. Insulin-sensitizing medications may be used as well.

Approximately 50–60 per cent of women with PCOS are obese. It has been shown that losing even 5 per cent of body weight can lead to an improvement in skin, regularity of menstrual cycles and decreased insulin levels. However, many women with PCOS experience difficulty losing weight, possibly due to high insulin levels promoting fat storage. High intakes of carbohydrates, especially refined carbohydrates (i.e. sweets, white bread, white rice, etc.) will quickly turn to sugar and cause elevated levels of insulin. Since high levels of insulin can cause a multitude of problems for women with PCOS, a low glycaemic index diet may be advised by medical experts.[35]

To sum up, although more research is needed it seems that a low glycaemic diet may play an important role in easing symptoms of

PCOS by helping to control insulin levels and promoting weight loss.

Peak performance

Long before the GI was recognized as a tool for weight loss, in addition to being used by diabetics it was also found to be useful for endurance athletes[36] who needed to boost their blood sugar levels both prior to and during an athletic performance.

The effect of glycaemic index on performance remains controversial, but it is thought that if athletes consume lower glycaemic index foods throughout the day they may not have a drop in blood sugar prior to training and/or competition, which will improve their performance. Conversely, consuming moderate to high glycaemic index foods during or after exercise is thought to promote muscle glycogen storage, which is good, since muscle glycogen is required for energy.

In summary, high glycaemic index foods may enhance performance in athletes and can be useful during and after workouts or competitions. Low glycaemic index foods may be helpful prior to sports activity. Insufficient research has been done to conclusively prove that there is a connection between carbohydrate consumption and athletic performance, but all the evidence[37] suggests that, whether you are an athlete or not, going on a glycaemic diet can boost energy, enhance stamina, prevent fatigue and help you perform at your maximum.

Children

Currently it is estimated that as many as 22 million children under the age of 5 are overweight. The statistics on the growing trend of obesity are alarming. Research shows that 70 to 80 per cent of obese children will become obese adults.

Parents of obese and overweight children often throw up their hands in nutritional confusion, not knowing what to feed their child or how to help, and studies have shown that the popular low fat, calorie-restricted approach is an exercise in futility, not just for adults but for children too. A recent study[38] found that when children and adolescents were placed on a reduced glycaemic load diet it had a greater effect on weight loss and insulin control than the standard reduced-fat diet.

In a nutshell, when it comes to helping children and adolescents lose or manage weight researchers have found that:

- Calorie restriction does not appear to work in the adolescent population. In fact, lack of calorie restriction was found to be a more positive approach for teenagers as it feels less like a 'diet'.
- Grainy foods (i.e. breads, pastas) promote weight gain by promoting excess secretion of insulin. In short, excess insulin = excess fat.
- The right type of fat, such as that found in nuts, seeds, olive oil and cold-water fish, is necessary for weight loss.
- Foods that are ranked lower on the glycaemic index and glycaemic load, such as fruits, non-starchy vegetables, nuts and dairy products, appear to promote weight loss and better insulin control.

As well as helping children to lose weight a glycaemic factor diet may also help boost a child's IQ. Research at Massachusetts Institute of Technology[39] found that children eating diets high in refined sugar had lower IQs than those raised on low GI diets. This is thought to be due to the reduced levels of brain boosting nutrients found in refined foods. High GI eaters of any age have been shown to be lacking in zinc, iron, folate and calcium.

Cognitive function

Researchers[40] at the Centre for Brain Health in the Department of Psychiatry at New York University School of Medicine have discovered that older individuals with unstable blood sugar levels are more likely to suffer from memory impairment and other cognitive difficulties.

In the study, published in the *Proceedings of the National Academy of Sciences*, researchers studied nondiabetic, non-demented middle-aged and elderly subjects to determine whether poor glucose tolerance is associated with reductions in memory and a smaller hippocampus, a brain area essential to learning and memory. The investigators studied the way glucose intolerance – a condition that precedes diabetes and is characterized by high blood sugar levels –

affected memory in 30 subjects (males and females). The researchers also studied the volume of the hippocampus, the part of the brain that plays a part in memory function.

The results of the study indicated that subjects with decreased glucose tolerance were more likely to suffer from decreased general cognitive performance, memory impairments and atrophy of the hippocampus.

As we've seen, glucose intolerance results when the body can't use insulin properly; insulin, of course, is the hormone that is responsible for driving blood sugar into body tissues. Researchers believe that glucose intolerance impairs memory because blood sugar fuels the brain, and if glucose remains in the bloodstream rather than being absorbed into body tissues, the brain operates less efficiently. It has long been known that diabetics often suffer from cognitive impairment, but this is the first study to show there is a link between the size of the hippocampus and the ability to control blood sugar levels in nondiabetics.

According to the study authors, this highlights the importance of blood sugar control for preserving and boosting cognitive function. For optimum brain function a low glycaemic load diet in combination with regular exercise is, therefore, highly recommended.

Depression

Abnormal fluctuations in your blood sugar can do more than set the stage for diabetes, heart disease, weight gain, poor concentration and poor health in general. They can also increase your risk of moodiness and depression because when high or low levels of sugar reach the brain, the result isn't just impaired memory but anger, irritability, slowed thinking and depression as well.

Your brain requires an even supply of blood glucose and requires the most glucose of any organ. In healthy people, blood glucose levels when fasting (between meals) are usually between 70 and 110 milligrams per decilitre (mg/dl). If levels fall too low or too high this can affect brain function and lead to poor concentration and mood swings – both early signs of adult-onset diabetes.

High GL diets create a quick mood boost but a mood crash follows soon after, leaving you feeling irritable and jittery. Studies[41] show that better glycaemic control with a low glycaemic diet prevents this roller-coaster effect and reduces the likelihood of depression and mood swings among both diabetics and nondiabetics.

Premature aging

As well as being critical for glucose metabolism and storage, insulin is also the hormone that helps other nutrients, such as vitamins, minerals, and amino and fatty acids, get inside the cells. While this is the normal mechanism that should occur, scientists are noticing an alarming increase in the breakdown of this metabolic process in people eating a diet high in sugar. If you aren't getting all the nutrients you need you won't be able to fight the free radical damage that causes wrinkles, lowered immunity, aches and pains and other signs of premature aging. For example, high GI diets decrease the amount of vitamin C you absorb from food by 25 per cent, and studies[42] have shown that people with high levels of vitamin C in their blood live up to six years longer than those with lower levels.

In many ways the low glycaemic load diet could be described as the ultimate anti-aging diet[43] in that it is a lifestyle of dietary habits that can keep wrinkles and premature aging at bay and lead you to longevity.

Lowered immunity

Sugar depresses the immune system.

In the 1970s researchers found out that vitamin C was needed by white blood cells so that they could counteract viruses and bacteria. Glucose and vitamin C have similar chemical structures; they compete with one another upon entering the cells. And what happens when the sugar levels go up? If there is more glucose around, there is going to be less vitamin C around. So when you eat sugar, think of your immune system slowing down to a crawl.

Here we are getting a little bit closer to the root of all disease. It doesn't matter what disease we are talking about, whether we are talking about a common cold or about cardiovascular disease, or cancer or osteoporosis, the root is always going to be at the cellular and molecular level, and more often than not insulin is going to have its hand in it, if not totally controlling it.

Because sugar is devoid of minerals, vitamins and fibre, and has such a deteriorating effect on the cellular, digestive and endocrine system, the majority of experts[44] agree that excessive sugar consumption is one of the leading causes of weakened immunity, poor health and degenerative disease in the Western world. Fluctuating blood sugar and insulin levels increase your risk not just of heart disease and diabetes but of practically every other age-related disorder – including obesity, cancer, hypertension, eye disease, fatigue, Alzheimer's, gallstones and arthritis – because they affect directly or indirectly virually every other disease process.

Box 1: Other ways a high sugar diet can damage your health and wellbeing

Studies[45] suggest that a diet high in sugar can negatively impact your health in the following ways. It can:

- upset the body's mineral balance;
- contribute to hyperactivity, anxiety, depression, concentration difficulties and crankiness in children – as well as contributing to eczema;
- cause kidney damage;
- lead to chromium and copper deficiency;
- interfere with absorption of calcium and magnesium;
- produce an acidic stomach;
- lead to periodontal disease;
- increase the risk of Crohn's disease and ulcerative colitis, and trigger gut dysbiosis;
- contribute to osteoporosis;
- cause food allergies;
- cause free radical formation in the bloodstream;
- cause toxaemia during pregnancy;
- overstress the pancreas, causing damage;
- cause atherosclerosis and hypertension;
- compromise the lining of the capillaries;
- cause liver cells to divide, increasing the size of the liver, and increase the amount of fat in the liver;
- cause hormonal imbalance and increase the risk of PMS and PCOS and fertility problems;
- increase bacterial fermentation in the colon;
- cause headaches, including migraines;
- increase blood platelet adhesiveness, which increases the risk of blood clots and strokes.

Some bad and good news

In addition to the conditions already mentioned in this chapter, research[46] also highlights other ways that a diet high in sugar can damage your health and wellbeing. Box 1 on page 61 lists some of these effects.

Clearly a diet high in sugar and refined carbohydrates, i.e. the typical Western diet, is bad news, but the good news is that you can do something about it. A glycaemic diet that controls blood sugar levels is proving to be a very successful dietary approach when it comes to boosting immunity and preventing, reversing and/or treating the majority of the health risks associated with a diet high in sugar. There is a great deal of evidence[47] to suggest that a glycaemic factor diet can promote rapid fat loss, increase energy, enhance mental clarity, lower blood pressure, slow aging, improve cholesterol and overall health, boost immunity, balance hormones and generate a feeling of euphoric wellness.

The new standard

Hopefully this chapter has given you plenty of reasons to eat a glycaemic factor diet. Here's a quick recap:

- If you cut out sugary foods from your diet you'll look younger.
- If you stick to a glycaemic factor diet you'll have more energy.
- Many exercisers find that they have better endurance on a glycaemic factor diet.
- A glycaemic factor diet can make you feel happier.
- Steady doses of glucose from low GL foods are good for your brain and can improve attention span and memory.
- A glycaemic factor diet helps keep your heart healthy.
- Reducing insulin levels can help acne and oily skin.
- Switching to a glycaemic factor diet can reduce the risk of diabetes.
- If you already have diabetes a glycaemic factor diet can help you control your condition more effectively.
- A glycaemic factor diet may even improve your vision.
- A glycaemic factor diet can cut the risk of ailments such as colds and flu.
- A glycaemic factor diet can reduce your risk of cancer.
- Women can dramatically benefit from a glycaemic factor diet as PMS and PCOS are associated with erratic blood sugar levels.

- Your fertility may improve by eating a low GI diet.
- A glycaemic factor diet can help you lose weight.
- A glycaemic factor diet can boost a child's IQ.
- A glycaemic factor diet may reduce the affects of premature aging and help you live longer.

Research[48] has clearly shown that the glycaemic factor diet isn't just a tool for the treatment of diabetics who want to maintain stable blood sugar; it has firmly established itself as the new standard for disease prevention, healthy eating, healthy weight loss and healthy living. Box 2 will help you to work out your glycaemic factor.

Box 2: What's your glycaemic factor?

If you'd like to know how at risk you are from health concerns due to a high glycaemic diet, answer the following and find out.

How often do you crave sugary snacks?

1 Once a day – usually around 3 or 4 p.m.	Score 2 points
2 When I'm feeling stressed or tired	Score 1 point
3 I don't get cravings at all	No points

Where are you most likely to gain weight?

1 Around my waist	Score 1 point
2 My hips and thighs	No points
3 Anywhere	No points

How many servings a day do you eat of the following?

1 White bread, bagels or rolls
2 White rice or rice cakes
3 Baked potatoes, mashed potatoes, chips, crisps
4 Cakes
5 Chocolate and sweets
6 Biscuits

Score 1 point for each serving

When you want a drink which are you most likely to choose?

1 Soft drinks or sweetened juices	Score 2 points
2 Alcoholic beverages	Score 2 points
3 Coffee or tea	Score 1 point
4 Water	No points

Which is your favourite fruit or which fruit do you eat the most?

1 Canned fruit in syrup	Score 2 points
2 Dried fruit	Score 2 points
3 Banana	Score 1 point
4 Apples, grapes or berries	No points

Do you get hungry between meals?

1 After breakfast – score 1 point
2 After breakfast and lunch – score 2 points
3 After every meal – score 3 points
4 Never – no points

Results

Over 10 points

You are eating a diet with a high glycaemic factor and may be suffering some of the symptoms. Constant hunger is a classic sign of blood sugar imbalance and sugar craving in the afternoon is a common sign too. If you're gaining weight around the middle the chances are your fat storage and distribution is being controlled by insulin. You will benefit greatly if you switch to a low glycaemic factor diet.

Between 5 and 9 points

Although your diet isn't definitely a high glycaemic factor one, there is still considerable room for improvement so you can enjoy all the health and weight management benefits that a low glycaemic diet can offer.

Less than 5 points

Congratulations! You are likely to be eating a low glycaemic factor diet, but perhaps there are still ways for you to maximize the benefits this healthy and satisfying way of eating has to offer. For example, perhaps you could be timing your meals better or combining your food choices with ingredients that lower your glycaemic factor even more.

Now that we've outlined the amazing health benefits of the glycaemic factor diet the next chapter will suggest simple and easy ways for you to incorporate it into a healthy eating plan that suits your lifestyle.

6

Getting started on your glycaemic factor diet

Now you know how much your health can benefit from the glycaemic factor diet, you'll probably be keen to get started. However, you may have a few reservations about changing your diet, especially if past attempts at dieting and weight loss failed. If this is the case here are some useful suggestions to help.

Start a food diary

You may find it helpful to keep a food diary and record what you eat and drink for a couple of days before making a change in your eating habits. This can be helpful because it will show you which areas of your diet most need improvement and when you are likely to crave food the most. You may also see a pattern emerging. Perhaps you eat a lot of refined carbohydrates, or perhaps you go for long periods without eating, or perhaps you eat a lot late at night. Becoming aware of your eating habits is the first step towards changing them.

Once you make the decision to begin your glycaemic factor healthy eating plan, write down the start date, your current size and weight and your health and weight loss goals. Then continue to write down everything you eat and drink and record your progress. A journal may seem like a waste of time but it really is worth creating one as researchers[49] have found that people who record their food intake daily lose more weight than those who don't. You'll learn a lot about your eating habits and lifestyle choices from your journal.

Harness your mental powers

Your ultimate success on a glycaemic factor diet doesn't just depend on your food choices, but on your mental choices.

Positive thinking isn't just a good idea when you begin the glycaemic factor diet – it's a necessity. Self-talk is a self-fulfilling prophecy because what you think you'll achieve will be exactly what you will achieve.

The first step in harnessing your mental power is to identify negative self-talk, such as . . .

Why should I succeed this time?
How can I possibly live without fast food?
I haven't got the discipline to stick to this.
If I lose weight I'll be sure to gain it again.
I've always hated vegetables.
Sweet food is such a comfort and a pleasure to me I'm not sure I can live without it.
Should I just accept being fat?
I eat out a lot so it's impossible for me to diet.
I haven't the time to think about what I'm eating.

You get the picture. Negative self-talk may sound logical but it is actually irrational and deceptive and only gives one view point: the negative view point. Just because you think something doesn't mean it is necessarily true. Yes, there's a chance you may not be able to live without fast food but there is also a chance that you will – so why not stress the positive instead of the negative? For every negative self-talk statement there is always an opposite, positive statement. You're in control of your thoughts, so why not choose the healthier and more positive option?

Although you may find it hard to believe, you can change virtually any thought you have. Once you have begun to identify the negative self-talk about your eating and your weight, the next step is to convert these statements into what you want to be true. For example, if you hate vegetables tell yourself that you can learn to like them. Tell yourself this often enough and your subconscious will start to believe it.

In your food diary or on a piece of paper, write down your biggest self-doubts, fears and objections about the glycaemic factor diet. Then underneath each one write the opposite positive. The main benefit of turning negative statements into positive ones is that you gain the power and momentum to reach your goals. Get your mind on your side and your chances of success will increase significantly.

Some people find affirmations helpful when it comes to making the necessary changes in self-talk. Affirmations are positive, motivating statements written in the present tense and they can be powerful tools that can help prove your inner self-doubts wrong. You can choose from the following or make up your own.

- I'm enjoying living and eating the glycaemic factor way.
- I'm enjoying the health benefits of the glycaemic factor way.

- I enjoy eating vegetables.
- I like to exercise.
- I enjoy planning, preparing and eating glycaemic factor meals.
- I feel good when I eat the low glycaemic factor way.

At least once a day, preferably more often, think or say each affirmation out loud. Set aside your doubts and just say them. You'll soon feel the flow of their power and eating the glycaemic factor way will become second nature.

One way of dealing with negative self-talk is to distance yourself from it. If you hear a negative voice yelling in your head it's hard to ignore it, but if you imagine that voice further away – so it comes from a distance, the little toe on your left foot, for example – it doesn't seem quite so overbearing. You might also want to change the tone of that voice and make it quieter or faster or make it sound like someone who makes you laugh, like Mickey Mouse. If you do that you may just find that what seemed overbearing and threatening has now become ridiculous. Why on earth would you listen to it or take it seriously? Try this next time you hear negative self-talk – it really can work.

Another technique is to talk back to your negative voices. Tell them how great you feel and how you are not going to listen to them any more. They'll soon give up. They can only stick around if you allow them to – because, remember, the only person who is in charge of the way you think is you. You and you alone have the power to get rid of them.

Your mental power is a terrific asset when it comes to healthy eating and losing weight. Positive thinking and affirmations can be great ways to harness the power of your mind and stay on track with your glycaemic factor diet.

When temptation strikes

The glycaemic factor diet isn't about being perfect all the time. It allows for the fact that you are going to slip now and again and make mistakes or over-indulge. You are human, after all, and no human is perfect.

Everyone makes mistakes, but try to think of these mistakes as lapses, not relapses. Lapsing is a normal part of changing but a relapse is going back to your old ways. The important thing is to understand why you lapsed – perhaps you got too hungry or didn't have time for breakfast or perhaps you simply forgot that from now on you are choosing to eat healthy things and feel and look great. If this happens, don't beat yourself up, just learn from your mistake.

But what about those times when it all feels too much and your craving for sweets, chocolate, etc. becomes overwhelming? Well, first of all you need to remember that the glycaemic factor diet allows you the odd indulgence. As mentioned earlier, as long as you eat healthily 80 per cent of the time you can still enjoy all kinds of foods. Sometimes, though, we crave a particular food we know isn't good for us, not because we really, really want it but because it has become a habit we find hard to break.

A habit is something you do repeatedly and automatically (without really thinking) and when challenged about the habit you find it difficult to change. Our brains have neural pathways and it takes an effort to remember to do things differently and to lay down new neural pathways. But with practice your brain will establish a new way of doing things, the old pathway will fade and a new habit, a new way of eating, will be formed.

Positive self-talk is a powerful weapon when temptation strikes and you find yourself looking at a sugary snack in the fridge, supermarket and restaurant out of habit. Here are some things you can say to yourself, either in your head or out loud if it helps, before you reach for the pastry, crisps, chocolates and so on:

Will this make me feel better or worse?
Seconds to eat but months on the hips.
I'm just not interested in feeling unhealthy any more.
I only eat healthy food not junk food.

This kind of statement or question can really stop you acting and eating out of habit because it helps you think about the consequences before you eat.

Getting motivated

Knowing that you need to improve your diet or lose weight isn't the same as making the decision to change your diet and/or lose weight. An important motivation-generating tool is visualization.

We tend to get what we focus on, so make sure you are focusing on what you want. Try this visualization exercise for yourself. It can be extremely powerful and motivating.

Think of yourself as the way you are now, the way you look and the way you feel. Now ask yourself: if you go on as you are now (eating too much unhealthy food, sitting down too much, drinking, etc.) what will your health and/or your figure be like in one year? Don't just think about your fatigue or mood swings: put as much feeling into the visualization as you can. You might want to go back to the previous chapter at this stage to remind yourself about the damaging effects of a high glycaemic factor diet.

Now ask yourself the same question again. This time travel forward two years. See yourself, hear yourself and feel what it would be like to be you – the way you'll be if you continue to neglect your diet and your health.

Repeat the process but this time fast forward five years, and then repeat again going forward ten years. Look at what you've become.

When you've seen about as much as you can stand of this unhealthy future, take a couple of deep breaths and turn the situation around. Go over the same questions again, but this time fast forward and see yourself the way you would be if you made the decision to eat and exercise for optimum health and wellbeing. What would you look and feel like if you made the changes you need to make right now? Just think how great you are going to feel when you have turned yourself around.

Are you motivated yet? You should be. If you aren't, just keep repeating this exercise over and over until it works.

Keep it realistic and simple

Many people give up on diets because they set unrealistic goals. Once you decide to make changes to your diet set yourself goals that are realistic and achievable.

Get the support of partners, family and friends and have strategies in place for when temptation strikes. Set yourself small achievable goals on the way towards your larger goal of better health and an ideal weight. For example, if you have four stone to lose, focus on losing that first half stone rather than the entire amount. Every time you achieve a milestone, give yourself a pat on the back.

Get yourself organized. If you were moving house or job you'd have an action plan, so do the same for a change in diet. It doesn't have to be anything complicated or long-winded – just decide what you are going to eat for a few days. Select the foods you want for breakfast, lunch, supper and snacks, write out a shopping list, go to the supermarket, buy the food, cook it, then enjoy it – nothing could be simpler.

Finally, as you begin the glycaemic factor diet, never forget that it is not a diet in the sense you may have understood the word before. It is not a short-term eating plan where you cut calories, restrict certain foods and feel deprived. It is a healthy, delicious, satisfying and permanent lifestyle change. Let's get started . . .

7

How do I follow a glycaemic factor diet?

The beauty of the glycaemic factor diet is that it is simple, straightforward and easy to follow. There aren't any complicated recipes or confusing dietary guidelines, so you can still follow the diet even if you have little time or inclination or ability to cook and prepare your food.

Make sure you eat three meals a day and two or three snacks, so that you never leave more than four hours between eating. If you go for long periods without eating you upset your blood sugar balance and this can cause fatigue and sugar cravings. You'll find plenty of ideas for breakfast, lunch, dinner and snacks in the next chapter. Alternatively you may decide to make up your own meals based on the glycaemic factor lists and guidelines in this book. If you eat out a lot you'll find plenty of advice to keep you on track with the glycaemic factor diet in Chapter 9.

Don't forget to watch your portion size. Supersizing is out, especially if you are watching your weight. A good rule of thumb is to feel satisfied after a meal and not bloated.

Most of us have foods that trigger overeating and these foods tend to be high GI foods, such as chocolate, crisps, white bread, biscuits and so on. The best way to deal with these trigger foods is to clear them out and keep them out of your house. Clearing out your fridge and food cupboard can be very liberating. It gives you the fresh start you need to create your new healthy eating plan.

Finally, try not to get so carried away with your healthy eating that you forget the importance of exercise. The evidence is beyond question: a glycaemic diet in combination with regular moderate exercise is the best thing you can do for your health. Aside from assisting in weight management (which was discussed in Chapter 4) regular exercise will:

- dramatically reduce your risk of heart disease, stroke, diabetes, cancer, high blood pressure and osteoporosis;
- boost your immune system;
- help you sleep better;
- help you beat sugar cravings;
- improve your mental wellbeing and boost your self-esteem.

Becoming more active will boost your health and wellbeing and help you lose weight if you have weight to lose. So in addition to making changes in your diet you also need to look at your day-to-day routine and see how you can become more active. Perhaps you could take the stairs instead of the lift. Perhaps you could cycle to work instead of getting the bus. Perhaps you could spend more time gardening. Perhaps you could chase the kids or your partner more! How about swimming, golf, yoga, dancing, sex, walking the dog? It doesn't matter what the activity is and you don't necessarily have to join a gym – as long as it gets you more active it will make a difference.

Box 3 has some useful tips on getting started with a regular exercise programme.

Box 3: Getting started with exercise

Often, the hardest part of getting into shape is taking the first step. Here is some simple advice to help you begin your journey.

To make physical improvements, you need to get more active than you are now. As a rule of thumb aim for around 30 minutes a day of moderate activity; if this isn't feasible go for three 10-minute sessions – it can be just as beneficial.

Exercise component 1: aerobic exercise

Aerobic exercise increases the health and function of your heart, lungs and circulatory system. For maximum effectiveness, aerobic exercise needs to be rhythmic, continuous and involve the large muscle groups. During aerobic exercise the aim is to gently increase your heart rate, not to strain it. You need to work harder than you normally would but not so hard that you get out of breath. Walking, jogging, cycling, swimming, aerobic dance and stair-climbing are examples of activities that use large muscle groups.

To achieve cardiovascular benefits, the American College of Sports Medicine (ACSM) recommends exercising 3–5 times per week (frequency) with a training heart rate of 60–85 per cent of your maximum (intensity) for 20–60 minutes (time).

Exercise component 2: strength training

Strength training is the process of exercising with progressively heavier resistance to build or retain muscle. Unless you

---

73

perform regular strength exercise, you will lose up to 0.25kg or 8oz of muscle every year of life after age 25. Muscle is a very active tissue with high energy requirements; even when you are asleep, your muscles are responsible for over 25 per cent of your calorie use. An increase in muscle tissue causes a corresponding increase in the number of calories your body will burn, even at rest.

To attain muscular fitness benefits, the ACSM recommends weight training two days per week, performing 1–3 sets of 10 repetitions of 8–10 different exercises. Don't panic, this doesn't mean you need to lift weights or join a gym – unless you want to. Some simple press-ups and sit-ups are fine, and there are plenty of books, magazines and videos that can guide you. If that doesn't appeal, just make sure you use your muscles more in your daily life; for example, carry your shopping bags, clean the car and so on.

Exercise component 3: flexibility

Flexibility is a critical element of an exercise programme but it is often overlooked. Stretching is important for a number of reasons: it increases physical performance, decreases risk of injury, increases blood supply and nutrients to the joints, increases neuromuscular coordination, reduces soreness, improves balance, decreases risk of low back pain, and reduces stress in muscles.

To improve your flexibility, gentle stretching exercises can be performed daily.

Choosing an exercise programme

The best choice is an activity that you enjoy enough to really pursue enthusiastically. Experiment with different forms of activity (cross training). Alternating new activities with old favourites will keep your enthusiasm high. Cross training also helps avoid injury due to repeatedly doing the same activity.

Begin slowly and gradually build

If you're just beginning an exercise programme, start slowly and gradually build. For example, participate in a cardiovascular activity (walking, aerobics, cycling, etc.) for 20 to 30 minutes, 3–5 times a week, and add strength training exercises (weight lifting, conditioning exercises) to your workout, twice a week. Schedule your strength training workouts with 48 hours' rest in between to allow your muscles to recuperate and repair after each workout.

If you attempt 'too much, too soon' it will lead to soreness, fatigue and maybe injuries. Work at your own level; start out slowly, and gradually increase duration and level of difficulty as your body progresses. Getting fit is not an overnight proposition, it's a lifestyle commitment. Don't expect immediate dramatic changes in your body shape or weight loss. Although changes are happening internally, most external benefits won't become visible for the first four to six weeks.

Staying motivated

Many people start an exercise programme with great enthusiasm only to drop out a few months or weeks or even days later. Here are some tips to help you stay motivated:

Find a fitness partner

Studies show that exercise adherence is generally greater if the family or a friend is included in the commitment to exercise. Find a walking partner, play tennis with your spouse, or go rollerblading with the kids.

Start an exercise log or journal

An exercise log or journal is an excellent way to chart your progress and provide motivation. Nothing beats the feeling of success as you read through your accomplishments. Exercise logs can take many forms: a calendar to record your workouts, a daily journal to record your feelings and goals, a computerized exercise log, or a log purchased at a bookstore. The key is to select a log or journal that fits your needs and provides you with the kind of information that is meaningful to you.

Throw out your scales

Ask yourself, 'How often has stepping on the scales in the morning ruined my day?' If your answer is 'often', consider whether or not you should give that little machine such power over you. The fact is that exercise should not revolve around a number on the scales. Exercise should be about making a commitment to your health and wellbeing; weight loss is a natural side effect of that commitment.

Schedule your workouts

Exercise must be a priority in order to establish it as a lifestyle practice. Make time for your workouts and schedule them on your daily calendar or planner. Make exercise non-negotiable: think of exercise as something you do without question, like brushing your teeth or going to work. Taking the lifestyle perspective will help you make exercise a habit.

Glycaemic factor food choices

Carbohydrates

When you start a glycaemic factor diet the biggest changes are likely to occur with your choice of starchy carbohydrates, i.e. bread, breakfast cereal, grains, pasta, potatoes and rice. This is simply because these foods are the ones our bodies convert most easily into glucose. These foods are also the ones we tend to eat the most.

There is no need to worry if you are one of the billions of people who love bread and pasta – the glycaemic factor does not ban these foods. Just make sure that you choose starchy carbohydrates that have a steadying effect on your blood sugar. The following guidelines will help you make the right carbohydrate food choices.

Bread

The more fibre a bread contains, the more likely it is to lower the GI. So go for added fibre or, better still, granary or wholegrain breads which can slow glucose conversion. Stoneground white or brown bread, barley, rye or pumpernickel bread, sourdough bread, fruit bread and soya bread are all good low GL breads to choose. Avoid white bread, rolls, baguettes, ciabatta and paninis made from finely ground or milled flour that hasn't broken down the glucose. (While trying to lose weight only consume one or two slices of bread a day, and if it causes bloating or you feel uncomfortable after eating bread try to get your fibre from other sources such as fruit and vegetables.)

Breakfast cereals

Breakfast is the most important meal of the day as research[50] has shown that regular breakfast eaters consume more nutrients, weigh less and have better concentration than those who skip breakfast. But a high GL breakfast cereal may be worse than having no breakfast at all as it is likely to trigger mid-morning food cravings for sugary snacks. The majority of breakfast cereals are high GL due to added sugar and honey and high levels of processing which make the starch bonds easy to break down and convert into sugar. The best breakfast cereal option is to go for high fibre and low sugar cereals such as bran or porridge oats. Muesli is a moderate choice but honey cereals, sugary cereals, wheat biscuits, flaked and puffed cereals (wheat, corn or rice) are best avoided.

Grains

Grains are nutritional superstars. They are high in essential vitamins and minerals, and because they are subject to minimal processing, grains also tend to be low GI. Increased use of grains is a characteristic of the glycaemic diet, but many of us simply aren't aware of the many different types of grains out there. Barley, couscous and quinoa have low GLs. Bulgar wheat and buckwheat have a moderate GL so use sparingly.

Grains are simple to cook; all you need to do is pop them into boiling water according to the instructions on the packet. They can be used instead of potatoes and rice. They can be used in flake form as a breakfast cereal or in flour form to make bread. They can be added to stews and soups to make a main meal. They can be added to salads to boost the fibre count and help you feel full. Fibre is a crucial part of a glycaemic factor diet and, generally, the more fibre a food has, the lower the GL.

Pasta

Pasta has a fairly low GI because of its protein and starch content which slows things down, but a moderate to high GL. This can be confusing, but not if attention is paid to portion size. Many of us eat much larger portions of pasta than are recommended. To estimate a portion more easily, a standard serving of pasta will fill half a cup. If you enjoy pasta don't overcook it as this raises the GL. Just boil it lightly with added olive oil and stick to eating all your pasta dishes al dente; serve as a side dish instead of making it your main meal.

When using pasta in recipes try to keep to no more than 100g in dry weight per person and use dried or fresh pasta (not tinned) with no added sugar. Noodles are usually made from wheat or rice and should be treated in the same way as pasta.

Potatoes

The good news is that some potatoes are okay on a glycaemic factor diet. New potatoes are fine, as are smaller immature potatoes that are not fully grown. Sweet potatoes and yams have a medium GL, so use only small quantities. Other root vegetables that have a low GL are swede, carrots, onions and garlic. The worst potato choices are chips, crisps, baked potatoes and instant mashed potatoes. (Corn products, such as tortilla chips, corn chips and so on, generally have a high glycaemic response so it's best to avoid them.)

Rice

Rice has an even higher GL than potatoes, pasta and bread, so it's best to substitute other food choices, such as vegetables, salad and couscous. If you want rice avoid any rice that takes less than 10 minutes to cook, such as jasmine rice or sticky rice, and choose wild rice or long grain rice such as basmati. And, as always, watch your portion size.

Aim to eat three to six servings a day of starchy carbohydrate foods such as bread, grains, pasta and rice. One serving is one slice of bread, a bowl of cereal or half a cup of rice or pasta.

Carbohydrate snacks

Biscuits, cakes, crisps, rice cakes, sweets and other sugary, salty or savoury snacks make up a large proportion of our calorie count. The bad news is that they either have a negative impact on our blood sugar levels or contain high levels of harmful fats called transfats. But this doesn't mean snacking is banned on a glycaemic factor diet. Quite the opposite – as mentioned earlier in this chapter, regular meals and snacks every two or three hours are needed to help keep blood sugar levels stable. You just need to choose the right kinds of snacks: those that are kind to your blood sugar levels.

Nuts, seeds, fruit, vegetable crudités, yogurt (as long as it has no added sugar) and even chocolate are all fine. If you want to eat chocolate, have two or three squares of high cocoa chocolate which has 70 to 85 per cent cocoa solids and less sugar. Chocolate is actually quite a healthy food as it contains high levels of antioxidants, as many as heart-healthy red wine. Remember, though, that added sugar-based ingredients like caramel will increase the GL, so stick to simple chocolate bars – particularly dark chocolate.

Fruits

It may surprise you but fruits are generally good food choices on a glycaemic factor diet: although they are sweet and are digested quickly, the main sugar in many fruits is fructose which is metabolized into glucose at a slow rate, helping to control insulin surges. This prevents sudden peaks in blood sugar that can cause blood sugar problems.

Aim to eat three to four servings of fruit a day. A serving is one piece of medium-sized fruit, a handful of grapes or two to three pieces of small fruit.

Low GL fruits
Apples
Apricots
Bananas (the GL increases when ripe so go for under-ripe green-flecked ones)
Blackberries
Blueberries
Cherries
Figs
Grapefruit
Grapes
Kiwis
Lemons
Limes
Mandarins
Mangoes
Melons
Nectarines
Oranges
Papaya
Pawpaw
Peaches
Pears
Pineapples

Plums
Raspberries
Strawberries
Tangerines
Watermelon

Dried fruits such as raisins, sultanas and prunes have a fairly high GL, but dried apricots, apples, strawberries and raspberries are much lower. Tinned fruits with added syrup and sugar should be avoided. The processing involved with canning fruit alters its make-up, increasing the rate at which glucose is created, and the syrup and sugars the fruit is canned in further raises the GL. Fruit juice also has a higher GL than the fruit it was extracted from as the fibre has been removed.

Vegetables

Most vegetables are low GL foods. This is because the actual amount of carbohydrate they contain is very small and in most cases they are not the types of carbohydrate to cause rapid rises in blood sugar. What's more, vegetables are high fibre foods and fibre is known to have a stabilizing effect on blood sugar. There are, however, exceptions – notably starchy root vegetables such as parsnips, swede and beetroot or sweet vegetables like pumpkin. This doesn't mean that parsnips and pumpkins are forbidden – no vegetable is banned on a glycaemic factor diet – it just means that portion size needs to be taken into account.

Don't forget that the GL of vegetables slightly increases when they are cooked or processed but the difference is so small that it won't affect your blood sugar levels significantly. In fact, some vegetables are more nutritious when they are cooked or frozen. For example, there is more betacarotene in cooked carrots than raw ones, as heat makes it easier for us to penetrate the tough cell walls and absorb the goodness inside.

Aim to eat at least five servings of vegetables a day. A portion of vegetables is three heaped teaspoons of cooked vegetables, a small bowl of salad or half a cup of raw vegetables.

Low GL vegetables

Artichoke
Asparagus
Aubergine
Avocado

Sugar-reduced baked beans
Black, butter, garbanzo, green, kidney, lima, haricot, pinto and soya beans
Bean sprouts
Broccoli
Brussels sprouts
Cabbage
Carrots
Cauliflower
Celery
Celeriac
Chickpeas
Collard greens
Corn on the cob
Courgettes
Endive
Kale
Kohlrabi
Leeks
Lentils
Lettuce
Mushrooms
Okra
Onions
Olives
Parsnip (moderate GL, so use sparingly)
Dried, green, yellow or split peas
Red, green, yellow or split peppers – plus hot peppers
Sugar-free pickles
Baby new potatoes
Pumpkin
Radish
Sauerkraut
Spinach
Yellow squash
Swede
Sweetcorn (moderate GL, so use sparingly)
Sweet potatoes (moderate GL, use sparingly)
Tomatoes
Watercress
Yams (moderate GL, use sparingly)

If you want to buy tinned vegetables go for those with no added sugar.

Salads are always a good and healthy choice, but watch the dressings as they can be high in fat and calories. Create your own dressings using vinegar, lemon juice, herbs and spices and olive oil. Studies[51] have shown that adding lemon juice or vinegar to a meal will reduce its GL.

Why are fruits and vegetables good for us?

All vegetables and most fruits are nutritional superstars. As well as aiding digestion and steadying blood sugar levels because of their fibre content, they are powerful sources of vitamins, minerals, phytochemicals (plant-based hormones) and antioxidants.

Antioxidants, such as vitamins A, C, and E as well as minerals like selenium, inhibit the harmful chemical process known as oxidation by neutralizing free radicals. Free radicals are the unstable, highly reactive and potentially harmful molecules formed in the body by a variety of sources: stress, digestion and smoking, to name but a few. Without intervention free radicals can wreak damage at a cellular level, accelerate the aging process and compromise the immune system. In addition to premature aging, conditions as varied as diabetes, heart disease, cancer, joint disease, asthma, senility and poor vision have all been linked to free radical damage.

Antioxidants help mop up free radical damage in our bodies, and making sure our diet is rich in them is a powerful form of preventative medicine. Vegetables and fruits are packed with antioxidants and the more we eat of them the more we strengthen our immunity against poor health and premature aging.

To make sure you get enough, aim to eat at least five portions of vegetables and three to four portions of fruit a day.

Protein

Pure protein foods such as meat, fish and poultry have no carbohydrate and therefore a low glycaemic factor. There are, however, some protein foods that contain both protein and carbohydrate and therefore a higher glycaemic factor.

Meat, fish, poultry and eggs

When buying meat, fish and poultry go for fresh produce rather than packaged. All fresh meats and fish are pure proteins that in their natural state are low glycaemic factor foods. Meats and fish that are coated in breadcrumbs or batter will have a higher glycaemic factor so choose natural, unprocessed lean cuts of meat and fresh fish where possible. Limit the amount of red meat you eat to one or two times a week as red meat tends to be high in unhealthy fats. Chicken and turkey and fish are fine alternatives to red meat, and quorn and soya are good vegetarian alternatives (and see Box 4). Oily fish, such as salmon, mackerel and sardines, are excellent protein choices. Eggs contain a wealth of nutrients and are fine as long as you don't eat more than one a day. Choose omega 3 eggs, which are high in healthy fatty acids, and boil or poach rather than frying.

Aim to eat up to two servings a day of protein – red meat no more than one or two times a week. If you are dieting watch your fat count. One serving is one egg or a portion of meat or fish about the size of a clenched fist.

Box 4: For vegetarians and vegans

Only a limited number of GI books cater for vegetarians, but the way of eating can easily be adapted to suit a vegetarian or vegan lifestyle, so long as the proportion of carbohydrates is kept low. When you look at the diets of most vegetarians and vegans, protein intake is very small. If you are a vegetarian it is very important that you get complete proteins in your meal. Here are some suggestions to help you do this:

- If you are the only vegetarian in your household, make sure you substitute pulses, beans, wholegrain cereals, dairy products, tofu or quorn instead of just leaving the meat part out of the meal. The best substitute for meat is soya protein and tofu.
- Bran cereals fortified with vitamins should be a regular part of your diet.
- Try to eat large portions of dark green leafy vegetables every day and drink a quarter of a pint of skimmed milk a

day to ensure you get your calcium. If you are lactose intolerant or vegan you can get your calcium in soya yogurts, milk and nut milks.

- Dried fruits, legumes and whole greens will ensure you get plenty of fibre and iron. Dark chocolate is a good source of iron too.
- Eat at least 30g of pulses, nuts and seeds every day for protein and essential fats.
- Eat at least one serving of low fat cheese or cottage cheese a day for protein and calcium – or a soya pattie or tofu portion.
- Eat at least four eggs a week if you're vegetarian.
- Choose margarine or butter fortified with vitamins D and E in a vegetarian spread. You can get vitamin D from sunlight as well, and vitamin E from nuts and seeds.
- If you are a vegan the risk of nutritional deficiencies is higher, and you need to seek expert advice from your doctor or a nutritionist if you decide to go on a glycaemic factor diet. Your biggest concern is to ensure adequate amounts of protein and vitamin B12. Soy protein, nuts, seeds, grains, pulses and vegetables are good sources of protein. Vitamin B12-fortified cereals are a good source of B12. You can also take a B-complex vitamin supplement which includes B12.

Dairy products

Dairy products aren't off limits on a glycaemic factor diet. They're a good source of protein and contain the sugar lactose which converts slowly, making dairy foods like milk, cheese and yogurt acceptable food choices. To lose weight and have a healthy heart, opt for low fat versions of dairy products. If you aren't lactose intolerant, skimmed or semi-skimmed is preferable to the full fat versions but try to limit yourself to a quarter of a pint a day. Unsweetened soya milk is also fine. Go for yogurt with no added sugar; Greek or bio yogurts are good choices. Cheese is also okay in small amounts but make sure the cheese is low fat. Low fat cottage cheese and cream cheese is also fine. If you must eat full fat cheese try to limit it to around 50g a day: 75g for low fat cheese.

Aim to eat one to two servings a day of dairy products – ideally low fat versions. One serving is about 55g or 2oz of cheese or 1 cup of milk or yogurt.

Nuts, seeds and legumes

Nuts and seeds have a low glycaemic factor and are a healthy choice if natural and unsalted and unsweetened. A good alternative snack to cakes and biscuits as they are less likely to stimulate food cravings, they are also vital sources of healthy fats that our bodies need. Research has shown that eating a handful of nuts a day can lower cholesterol levels and aid weight loss.

Nuts like peanuts, walnuts, cashews and brazil nuts and seeds like pumpkin, hemp and sunflower can make a delicious snack or be sprinkled over salads and other vegetable or meat dishes. Bear in mind, too, that spreads and dips and oils made from nuts and seeds, such as peanut butter and sunflower oil, will have a lower glycaemic factor than butter or margarine. If you are watching your weight, nuts and seeds are very high in calories so they should be kept to a minimum: no more than a handful a day.

Legumes

Legumes are a valuable source of protein, fibre, calcium, potassium, magnesium, iron and B vitamins. A diet that is rich in regular servings of legumes, or beans and pulses, has been shown to help lower cholesterol, balance blood sugar levels and, according to some researchers,[52] can help boost immunity, health and wellbeing. With the possible exception of broad beans (fava beans), all beans and pulses have a low glycaemic factor due to their high fibre content which slows sugar conversion.

Most of us don't eat enough of these healthy, low calorie foods so try to eat more. Healthy choices include: sugar-free baked beans, black beans, butter beans, chickpeas, haricot beans, kidney beans, mung beans, lentils, soya beans, split peas and products made from beans and pulses such as hummus and soups. Adding beans to soups, salads and casseroles will slow down the digestion of the meal.

Aim to eat one to three servings a day and oils made from these one or two times a day. One serving is half a cup of beans, a small handful of nuts and seeds or two tablespoons of oil.

Good fats versus bad fats

Most foods that are high in fat are relatively low on the glycaemic factor because fat does not raise blood sugar levels significantly. However, a diet that is too high in fat can be damaging to your health and your waistline, so a glycaemic factor diet needs to include the right kinds of fats.

As mentioned previously, fat is essential for health and wellbeing. Your body uses fat for energy, to process vital nutrients that keep your skin, hair, brain, eyes and bones healthy and to create healthy cells and hormones which regulate your mood and your appetite. In short, without enough fat in your body you won't look or feel good; but you need to ensure you are getting the right type of fat.

There are four types of fat: saturated, monosaturated, polyunsaturated and hydrogenated, also known as transfats (hydrogenated fats are made when vegetable oils are processed through extreme heat). Research[53] suggests that saturated and hydrogenated fats have been linked to obesity, heart disease and cancer. On a glycaemic factor diet you should aim to choose foods that have a low glycaemic factor – but when these foods contain fat you should pick those high in healthy fats rather than unhealthy ones.

So make sure you avoid unhealthy saturated fats – found in butter, meat and full fat dairy products – and unhealthy transfats – found in hard margarines, cakes, biscuits and other highly processed foods. Instead, go for healthy monosaturated fats – found in olives, nuts, seeds, avocados and the oils obtained from them – and healthy polyunsaturated fats – found in oily fish such as trout, salmon, mackerel and herring.

Studies[54] show that people who use olive oil regularly tend to have lower cholesterol levels and better health in general. So wherever possible use olive oil in your cooking and to make up your own dressings, and go for olive oil spreads.

Studies[55] also show that an essential fat called omega 3 can help fight and prevent heart disease, cancer, depression, diabetes, hyperactivity and other diseases, and it's important to make sure you include enough in your diet. Flax seeds, hemp seeds and walnuts are good sources, as is fish oil. So eat more fish like salmon, trout, mackerel and sardines, as well as plenty of white fish. Fish oil supplements, or flax or hemp seed oil if you're a vegetarian or vegan, are highly recommended.

Making sure your diet is rich in healthy fats and avoiding

unhealthy fats is the key to good health. A glycaemic factor diet makes this easy to achieve, as generally foods that are high in unhealthy fat are also high in sugar. However, just to make sure you are eating the right kinds of fats, always read food labels, choose low fat wherever possible and avoid frying.

Salt

Another health hazard is a diet too high in salt. Many of us eat far more salt than is recommended. The recommended intake is 5–6g a day but most of us eat 12g or more. Too much salt increases the risk of high blood pressure, a major cause of strokes and heart attacks, and is also linked to problems such as fluid retention, asthma and stomach cancer.

Most of us just aren't aware of how much salt we are eating because it is a hidden ingredient in so many processed and packaged foods. Salt is typically listed as sodium on food labels – to find out how much salt is actually in something, multiply the sodium amount by 2.5.

To lower your salt intake, get out of the habit of automatically sprinkling your food with salt, and as much as possible avoid processed foods and go for fresh, unprocessed ingredients instead. Reduce the amount of salt you use in cooking by experimenting with alternative seasonings such as herbs, spices, vinegar and lime and lemon juice.

Sugar and sugar substitutes

You probably don't need reminding at this stage that sugars are a flashing red light area and should be avoided as much as possible on a glycaemic factor diet. Gradually reduce the sugar used in tea and coffee and always check food labels for the sugar content. As well as sugar, brown sugar and corn syrup, other names that are used on ingredient labels include: sucrose, glucose, dextrose, fructose, maltose, modified food starch, natural sweeteners, lactose, sorbitol, mannitol, honey, corn syrup, corn syrup solids, high fructose corn syrup, molasses and maple syrup. Here's a list of the ones you should definitely avoid:

• Sucrose, or table sugar, from sugar cane or sugar beet, consists of two simple sugars, glucose and fructose. It is about 99.9 per cent pure and sold in either granulated or powdered form.

- Raw sugar consists of coarse, granulated crystals formed from the evaporation of sugar cane juice. It is best avoided because of impurities.
- Brown sugar consists of sugar crystals contained in a molasses syrup with natural flavour and colour. Some refiners make brown sugar by adding syrup to refined white sugar. It is 91 to 96 per cent sucrose.
- Turbinado sugar is raw sugar that goes through a refining process to remove impurities and most of the molasses. It is edible if processed under proper conditions; however, some samples in the past contained trace contaminants.
- Invert sugar is a mixture of glucose and fructose. Invert sugar is formed by splitting sucrose in a process called inversion. This sugar prevents crystallization of cane sugar in confectionery making.
- Icing sugar, also called confectioner's sugar or powdered sugar, consists of finely ground sucrose crystals mixed with a small amount of corn starch.
- Honey is an invert sugar formed by an enzyme from nectar gathered by bees. Honey contains fructose, glucose, maltose and sucrose. Honey contains only trace amounts of vitamins and minerals. One would have to eat large quantities before any nutritional benefit would be received.
- High fructose corn syrup (HFCS) is a sweetener made from corn starch. The amounts of fructose vary with the manufacturer. An enzyme-linked process increases the fructose content, thus making HFCS sweeter than regular corn syrup.
- Corn syrups, produced by the action of enzymes and/or acids on corn starch, are the result of splitting starch. Three major producers contain 42 per cent, 55 per cent and 90 per cent fructose. Dextrose comprises most of the remainder.
- Levulose, or fructose, is a commercial sugar much sweeter than sucrose. Its sweetness actually depends on its physical form and how it's used in cooking.
- Dextrose, or glucose, is also known as corn sugar. It's commercially made from starch by the action of heat and acids, or enzymes. It is sold blended with regular sugar.
- Lactose, or milk sugar, is made from whey and skimmed milk for commercial purposes. It occurs in the milk of mammals. The pharmaceutical industry is a primary user of prepared lactose.
- Sorbitol, mannitol, malitol and xylitol are sugar alcohols or

polyols. They occur naturally in fruits and are produced commercially from such sources as dextrose. Xylitol is a sugar alcohol made from a part of birch trees.

Are any of these sugars better than the others? No. Forget the fancy names. The bottom line is 'sugar is sugar'. Brown sugar is sucrose, just like white sugar. Brown sugar may have had less processing than white, but it still has little nutritional value. Raw sugar is also sucrose, just like white sugar. Raw sugar is just less refined than white sugar, but again this does not offer any nutritional value. Sugar in any form is high in calories and low in nutrients. The body uses it the same way, no matter what the source.

Low fat products often have the fat replaced by sugar and even salty or savoury food choices can have sugar added to them, so be alert to that. To monitor your sugar intake always ensure you read food labels as sugar is a cheap ingredient used in the majority of processed foods. As a rule of thumb, if sugar is listed within the first five ingredients on a food label, choose an alternative.

If you need a sugar substitute the best natural sweetener you can use is fruit or fruit juice. Fructose, which is a natural sugar occurring in fruit, probably has the lowest glycaemic response, but do use it sparingly. The odd teaspoon of honey is fine too. When it comes to artificial sweeteners, it is probably best to avoid them as a number of studies[56] have suggested that they aren't good for your health. You could try the herbal alternative stevia, which is sweet tasting, low glycaemic and calorie free.

Drinks

It isn't just food that interferes with your blood sugar levels – drinks can too. Choosing low glycaemic factor drinks is just as important as choosing low glycaemic factor foods.

Lemon and orange squash, cola, fizzy drinks, sports drinks and beer are all high in sugar and should be limited or avoided. Some studies[57] have also shown that excessive amounts of coffee can increase the chance of cells becoming insulin resistant, so ideally on a glycaemic factor diet you should limit the coffee you drink to no more than one or two cups a day.

The problem with coffee, and with tea and fizzy drinks, is that many of us become addicted to the caffeine – and when we stop drinking it we get headaches. To get around this give your body time to adjust: wean yourself off excessive caffeine consumption slowly by cutting back or watering down your coffee over a period of several weeks, rather than days.

Low fat milk, fruit and herbal tea are acceptable on a glycaemic factor diet. When it comes to juice, apple, orange, pear, grapefruit, peach, pineapple and cranberry pure fruit juices are also acceptable. Alcoholic spirits, such as gin and whisky, have a moderate glycaemic response but should be avoided as they are linked to health problems. Red wine is better than white wine and spirits as it contains antioxidants which are good for your heart.

The healthiest and most refreshing drink, however, has to be water. Most of us simply don't drink enough water even though it is essential to life. The nutrients from our food are transported around the body by water, we need water to remove waste products, water regulates body temperature and most chemical reactions in the body need water. If you don't drink enough water you can feel tired, constipated, nauseous and may even get headaches. To keep the fluid balance right in our bodies most of us need around six to eight cups or glasses of water, preferably bottled or filtered water, each day. If it's hot or we have been sweating a lot because of strenuous exercise we need more than usual to stay cool.

If you don't like drinking water try spicing it up by adding a slice of lemon or orange, or perhaps you could dilute unsweetened fruit or vegetable juices. Caffeinated drinks, such as tea and coffee, aren't a good idea because they are diuretic and can cause fluid loss. And don't forget that fruits and vegetables consist of 90 per cent water.

Water is absolutely essential so make sure you drink plenty. One way to ensure that you drink enough is to fill a jug or bottle of water with your targeted amount of water and drink it throughout the day. Take it with you in the car or to work or keep it nearby when you are reading or doing other activities. If the container is empty by bedtime you've achieved your goal.

8

Designing your glycaemic factor diet

If you're looking for glycaemic set menus, meal plans, recipes and eating schedules there are plenty on the market (some of the most popular were mentioned in Chapter 4). If, on the other hand, you want the flexibility to design your own glycaemic factor diet you'll find lists of low glycaemic breakfasts, lunches, dinners and snacks in this chapter.

Select what you want from the lists below and refer to the shopping guidelines later in the chapter before you buy your ingredients. Just make sure that you watch your portion size, that you don't leave more than a few hours between meals and snacks, and that you eat a balanced and varied diet according to the guidelines given in previous chapters. Once you get used to the glycaemic menu options listed below and feel confident enough to go it alone, you can use the advice in this book and start devising your own meal plans.

Low glycaemic factor breakfasts

Tip: breakfast is the most important meal on a glycaemic factor diet – so never miss it!

Reduced-sugar baked beans on toasted low GL bread
Boiled eggs with low GL bread
Sugar-free jam or marmalade on low GL bread
Scrambled eggs on low GL toasted bread
Low GL toasted bread with cream cheese, ham and tomato
Grated cheese on toasted low GL bread with a slice of tomato
Poached eggs on low GL toasted bread
Sardines on low GL toasted bread
Low GL toasted bread with peanut butter
Large slice of watermelon
Low GL fruits topped with a tablespoon of Greek yogurt
Mushroom omelette
Smoked salmon or tuna omelette
Bran cereal with skimmed milk

91

Cheese or bacon and tomato omelette
Grilled bacon with poached egg and grilled tomatoes
Fruit smoothie made with skimmed or soya milk and low GL fruits
Fresh fruit with almonds
Grilled bacon and tomatoes
Cold lean ham and sliced pear
Plain yogurt and oat-based cereal bar
Muesli
Oat porridge with fresh strawberries

Low glycaemic factor lunch or dinner

Tip: it's always best to go for a light dinner and a more substantial lunch – and, remember, don't ever be tempted to skip either meal.

Cottage cheese salad with vinegar and olive oil-based dressing
Egg salad
Fish fingers, poached egg, reduced-sugar baked beans
Lentil soup
Celery soup
Carrot and coriander soup
Asparagus soup
Tomato soup
Three-bean soup (French, kidney and haricot)
Medium sweet potato and side salad with olive oil dressing
Bacon and salad sandwich on low GL bread
Low fat cottage cheese and tomato sandwich on low GL bread
Poached eggs, bacon and tomato
Tuna or oily fish with salad
Smoked salmon pâté with basmati rice
Prawn salad
Any poached fish with salad and olive oil dressing
Chicken or turkey with salad and olive oil and vinegar dressing or
low fat mayonnaise
Cheese and tomato salad
Egg salad
Mozzarella cheese and tomato slices with balsamic vinegar dressing
Wholemeal pasta with pesto and walnuts
Lentil, chicken and bacon salad
Tomato, mozzarella and olive salad with a small wholemeal pitta
Falafels and salad

Grilled herring with oatmeal coating and apple sauce
Fish cakes with fresh tomato sauce
Baked potato with reduced-sugar baked beans
Pearl barley risotto with peas
Grilled salmon fillet with chickpea and parsley puree
Chicken or vegetable curry with basmati rice

Useful tips:

Home-made soups are always best, or look for soups that have no added sugar, potatoes, rice, pasta or croutons.

A teaspoon of tomato or brown sauce is fine to add to your cooking or meals.

Make your own baked beans with cannellini beans and fresh tomato sauce to avoid the sugar high of tinned baked beans.

Avoid ready-made sauces, pickles and chutneys as they are high in sugar and flour. Home-made sauces, pickles and chutneys with glycaemic friendly ingredients are best.

Vinegar, lemon and lime mixed with olive oil is always a good choice as a dressing, but you could also experiment with lemongrass, ginger, garlic and other herbs and spices mixed with natural yogurt.

Low glycaemic factor desserts

Tip: best option is always a low glycaemic fruit, but if you fancy the occasional treat:

Banana fool with Greek yogurt
Baked apple filled with sultanas and cinnamon
Vanilla ice cream with strawberries
Pears cooked in red wine and cinnamon
Stewed apricots with blueberries
Halved peaches with toasted almonds
Baked egg custard
Chocolate sponge pudding
Low fat muffins
Blueberry and apple crumble
Wild berries with frozen yogurt

Low glycaemic factor snacks

Tip: remember, a mid-morning snack, a mid-afternoon snack and perhaps a snack before bedtime are not optional extras but essential parts of a glycaemic factor diet.

Fruit smoothie made from fresh fruits blended with ice
Cappuccino made with water and skimmed milk
Two oat biscuits and a slice of low fat cheese
A small handful of olives
A small cup of low fat cottage cheese with dried apricots
One slice malt loaf
Plain yogurt with fresh blueberries, strawberries or raspberries
Two squares of dark chocolate
One serving of fruit or a bunch of grapes
A handful of nuts and/or seeds, such as almond, brazil nuts and pumpkin, linseed and sunflower seeds
Crudités with hummus
Cut-up vegetables with dip
Low fat blueberry muffin
Hard-boiled egg
Slice of pumpernickel rye bread
A small baked yam topped with two tablespoons of plain yogurt
A small handful of dried apricots and cranberries
Two meat and cheese rollups – use a thin slice of meat and cheese and a lettuce leaf; secure with a tooth pick
Plain whole fruit with a cup of herbal tea

Contrary to popular opinion, cereal and snack bars are not generally a healthy choice. Even the natural ones sold in health food stores are high in sugar and are best avoided.

Low glycaemic factor drinks

Coffee with no added sugar or syrup
Tea with no added sugar
Herbal tea
Bottled water
Sugar-free smoothies
Soya milk
Vegetable juices
Fruit juices
Diet drinks with no caffeine and added sugar
The odd glass of red wine
The odd glass of dry white wine
The odd glass of reduced carb lager

Glycaemic factor shopping and cooking guidelines

Restock your fridge and shelves with healthy, nutritious ingredients fit for the happier, healthier and slimmer you. If you've followed the advice in this book so far, your shopping habits may already be changing. You'll be reading food labels and noticing how many processed and high glycaemic factor foods there are in many of the foods you may have eaten on a daily basis.

A diet high in nutrients and low in sugar, unhealthy fat, additives and preservatives is the key to good health. But supermarkets can be confusing with so many different types of foods, labels and brands. In this section you'll learn some simple guidelines to help you shop for glycaemic factor weight loss and good health. Don't panic – although you may find yourself buying new and different kinds of foods, you'll find the new way of shopping just as easy as before.

When you are ready to go shopping, first make sure you aren't hungry – because if you are, you're more likely to fill your trolley with easy to prepare and eat high glycaemic factor foods! You may also find it helpful to sit down and plan which fresh, natural and low glycaemic factor ingredients you want to stock your cupboard, fridge and freezer with. As you review this list, here's what will happen. You'll find that most of the foods you buy from now on are available on the outside perimeter of the store, in the fruit and vegetable section or frozen food section. With the exception of spices, olive oil, vinegar and the odd item here and there you won't need to walk down the food aisles packed with carbohydrate and sugar-rich foods any more.

Note: It's always a good move to choose food that is organically produced as it has fewer chemicals and additives and tends to be less processed.

Cupboard

Glycaemic factor beans and pulses (see p. 85 and Box 5)
Low glycaemic factor bread, for example stoneground bread
Wholegrain pasta
Couscous
Basmati rice
Dried apricots
Extra virgin olive oil
Ground almonds – to take the place of flour in baking
Herbs and spices of your choice – to take the place of salt and sugar

Nut oils, such as walnut and macadamia
Cold-pressed oils such as flaxseed, soybean, sunflower and canola oils
Pesto
Reduced-sugar baked beans
Seeds – linseeds, pumpkin seeds, sunflower seeds, hemp seeds, sesame seeds
Sundried tomatoes in olive oil
Tinned fish, tuna and sardines
Traditional oats
Unsalted nuts – almonds, hazelnuts, walnuts, pecans, pinenuts, peanuts
Bran cereal fortified with vitamin B12
Muesli
Vinegar – balsamic, red and white wine or flavoured vinegar
Glycaemic factor grains, for example pearl barley
Sweet potatoes, new potatoes or yams

Box 5: Beans and pulses

Avoid canned beans with salt or preservatives and frozen beans. Choose instead beans cooked without animal fat or salt. Why? Beans are a fantastic source of nutrients that can help reduce cholesterol and balance your blood sugar, but their nutritional value can be depleted if they are canned or cooked in fat and salt. Canned beans are more likely to be high in toxic preservatives and additives, and beans cooked in saturated fats and salt can counteract the cholesterol and glucose lowering effect of the beans and increase the risk of weight gain, heart disease, fluid retention and high blood pressure.

Beverages

Avoid alcoholic drinks, coffee, cocoa, pasteurized and/or sweetened fruit juices and drinks, sodas and teas. Choose instead herbal teas, fresh (preferably organic) fruits and vegetables and fruit juices, mineral or distilled water. If possible choose glass bottles. There is always a certain amount of residue that dissolves into a drink from the lining of a can or from a plastic bottle, so it's always best to choose glass bottles.

Fridge

Non-fat cottage cheese
Unsweetened yogurt, Greek-style yogurt
Skimmed milk or soya milk
Half fat cheese
Olive oil-based spreads
Small pot of single cream or vanilla ice cream
Organic free range eggs – these won't contain the toxic hormones and antibiotics pumped into factory-produced eggs
Ready-made soups that are low in fat and salt
Small bar of dark chocolate

Fruit

Choose from the glycaemic factor fruit list on p. 79.

Avoid canned, bottled or frozen fruits with sweeteners added. Choose instead all fresh, frozen, stewed or dried fruits without sweeteners or additives. Fruits are high in essential fibre, vitamins, minerals and antioxidants. It is always best to eat them fresh because when they are processed or juiced their nutrient and fibre content decreases and their sugar and additive content increases.

And remember not to buy too much fruit, as fresh fruit doesn't stay fresh for long. As far as fruit and vegetables are concerned it's always best to buy small amounts more often. Don't forget to add lemons and limes to your list; not only do they add a tangy flavour to dishes, they can also lower the overall glycaemic factor of your meals.

Vegetables

If you're like most people you've probably eaten the same vegetables for years. Now that you need to eat at least five servings of vegetables a day it is time to shop this section with new eyes.

Select your vegetables and purchase fresh and frozen. Fresh vegetables keep about a week in the fridge, frozen keep much longer. Frozen vegetables are a good back-up in case you run out of fresh during the week and are a good choice because they are frozen at optimum ripeness. Fresh produce is sometimes harvested weeks before it arrives at the greengrocer's shelves and may have lost important nutrients in transit.

Meat and fish

All meats and fish have a low glycaemic factor. Choose lean meats that are as natural as possible without any additives. Try to balance the amount of red and white meat you buy and buy lots of fish. When buying fish avoid all fried fish, shellfish, salted fish, anchovies, herring and other fish that is canned in salt and oil, and choose instead all freshwater white fish, salmon, boiled or baked fish, water-packed tuna.

Freezer

Although it's always best to eat foods that are fresh, frozen – preferably organic – vegetables and fruit that are salt, sugar and additive free are great standbys as they retain their nutritional quality.

Frozen fish, chicken and meats in their natural states are also low glycaemic. Natural is always best on a glycaemic factor diet so avoid the battered or breadcrumbed processed products.

Now and again when life is really hectic you may need to eat something that only takes a few minutes to cook. If this is the case the odd pre-packed frozen meal won't hurt as long as you always glance at the label to ensure the ingredients are relatively glycaemic factor friendly and that the list of ingredients isn't too long. Some ready meals will be quite high in fat but the light options will be high in sugar and additives, so be careful.

Glycaemic factor cooking guidelines

Cooking based on the glycaemic factor is more balanced and healthy and is actually easier than other ways of cooking; all you'll really be doing is substituting higher glycaemic factor foods with lower ones.

The following glycaemic factor cooking basics will help you:

- About a quarter of each meal needs to be protein. Think eggs, meat, fish, poultry, cheese or soya for breakfast, lunch or dinner.
- Add in vegetables for lunch and dinner and if possible breakfast. Vegetables should comprise about half of your meal.
- The final quarter of the meal should consist of yams, legumes, fruit, dairy and wholegrain pasta or rice.
- A low glycaemic cookbook might be a wise investment to give you a feeling for ingredients and preparation methods.

- Cook with olive oil.
- As much as possible, include raw fruits and vegetables and fresh ingredients in your cooking and avoid processed ones. Processed foods are not only less nutritious, they have been shown to increase glycaemic load.[58] Raw foods are packed with life-enhancing enzymes and nutrients, have enough protein and are low in fat as well as slow-releasing carbohydrates that boost energy and fibre that improves digestion. (Perhaps the most energizing and beneficial raw food choice you can make is sprouts. Sprouts refer to the seeds of legumes and grains that have been germinated for three to five days into small plants. Each sprouting seed has enough nutritional and life force to grow into a healthy plant, and that is why they have more nutritional activity than any other raw food – because they are still in the process of growing.)
- Avoid cooking at extreme temperatures and keep cooking to the absolute minimum. The more a food is cooked, especially vegetables, the higher its glycaemic load. Proteins are also not spared by cooking. When proteins are cooked too much the protein itself is actually destroyed, rendering it at least useless and at worst harmful. Cooking generally causes nutrient loss which compromises the overall immune system and leads to fatigue and weight gain. This doesn't mean you shouldn't cook food at all. Our systems couldn't handle an all raw diet and certain foods, such as eggs, meats and fish, are extremely dangerous to eat when raw and need to be cooked thoroughly. You must still eat cooked food but just try to balance it with more raw: perhaps a 50–50 ratio of raw to cooked food.
- When you do cook, cook gently, and for longer if need be, at a lower heat, letting your food simmer or steam lightly. When cooking fruits and vegetables it is best to warm them rather than vigorously cook them. (A good trick when making soup is to heat the soup and then at the last minute add some raw vegetables which are just warmed by the soup broth.) Steaming is the best way to cook vegetables. Stir frying is a good way to cook fish, meat and vegetables. Poaching is a good way to cook eggs and fish. Roasting is the best way to cook meat, since other methods such as frying use too much fat and should always be avoided. Boiling isn't the best way to cook vegetables as the nutrients tend to leach into the liquid during the cooking process. If you do boil vegetables keep the water to add to soups and casseroles. (Please

note that some ingredients, such as dried beans and pulses, must be boiled in plenty of unsalted water until they are fully cooked.)

- When cooking, avoid dishes that involve the addition of creamy and rich sauces and salt. Use herbs and spices instead.
- As for microwaving, we don't have any clear idea of the effects yet and we do not know what molecular changes may be happening to the food when cooked. Best to limit as much as you can.

9

The glycaemic factor and children

Preparing meals for a partner or family members can be challenging even without the glycaemic factor to consider, but as the glycaemic factor diet will improve everyone's health there is no need to apologize for the foods you buy, eat and prepare. In the first few weeks you may encounter resistance to the change in menu and it might be a good idea to keep a few high glycaemic factor snacks on hand. However, once your partner and/or family discover that the glycaemic factor diet is satisfying, delicious and not restrictive (remember the 80–20 rule), if you are patient everyone's nutrition and health will improve because yours has.

The hardest members of the family to win over are most likely to be children who may have grown accustomed to a diet high in fat and quickly digested carbohydrates, but helping our children eat well is perhaps one of the most important things we can do for them.

Many children's favourites, such as nuggets, chips, crisps, sweets, sugary cereals, instant mash and so on, have high glycaemic values and it is easy to overconsume calories with these foods and put on weight. In contrast, studies[59] have shown that when children are fed low glycaemic factor foods like fruits, vegetables and porridge, not only do they stop overeating and feel more satisfied but body mass index and body weight decrease significantly.

A horrifying 13 per cent of UK and 19 per cent of US youngsters are now classified as obese while many more are overweight. This adds up to a serious health problem, because those extra pounds increase the risk of heart disease, high blood pressure, diabetes, gallstones, osteoporosis, fertility problems, cancer and depression later in life.

Action is clearly needed – but how do you tackle or prevent childhood obesity without causing low self-esteem, food cravings or eating disorders? The answer is to incorporate more low glycaemic factor foods into your child's diet and to tailor your approach to your child's age. Here's how it's done.

Incorporating low GI foods into your child's diet

A healthy diet for a child supplies all the nutrients needed for growth and development. It also allows for varied and interesting meals, accommodates a child's routine, satisfies a child's appetite, encourages good eating habits and maintains a healthy body weight.

If you are already eating plenty of whole grains, fruits and vegetables, drinking plenty of water and including low fat protein in your diet from fish, lean meat and dairy products, the chances are your child will imitate you. If, however, your child has grown accustomed to high glycaemic carbohydrates, sugar and fast food, when you start making changes to their diet and substituting high glycaemic factor food choices with low glycaemic factor food choices you are bound to encounter resistance.

Children always dislike new foods and it is entirely normal for them to reject them. However, repeated exposure to new foods in an upbeat environment will encourage them to experiment. But you will have to be patient and persevere. Be prepared; it may take ten or more times before a child finally accepts it.

It isn't necessary to make your children eat low glycaemic factor foods alone. On the contrary, balanced meals usually consist of a variety of foods and eating low glycaemic factor foods with high glycaemic factor foods produces a medium glycaemic factor.

It's also important to bear in mind that children are natural grazers. They actually prefer to have several meals and snacks throughout the day and it is a mistake to force them to eat everything on their plate as this can encourage overconsumption. Children have small stomachs so let them stay in tune with their appetite and eat according to it. So long as the meals and snacks you offer your kids are low glycaemic and nutritious, appetite is the best measure of how much they need to eat.

Tailoring your approach to your child's age

Preschool

Up to the age of 5 or 6 it's normal for children to accumulate more fat on their arms and legs than their bodies. Dimpled thighs are not a sign of being overweight.

Dos:

- Do breastfeed if you can. Babies breastfed up to six months are less likely to become obese in childhood than formula-fed children. But if you can't or don't want to breastfeed don't beat yourself up – the most important thing at this stage for your child is a happy and loving mum.

- Do watch how you wean your child. There is no need to add chips, butter or junk food. Now is a great time to introduce fruits and vegetables along with a baby's normal milk.
- Do make sure you never force your child to eat when he or she is full. Most children stop eating naturally when full but if a child does overeat and vomit, teach him to stop eating before he feels full.
- Do avoid giving sweets until at least the age of 2. Satisfy a sweet tooth with fresh and dried fruit, yogurt and low sugar muesli bars.
- Do set a good example. Children learn their eating habits from their parents. If you snack on high glycaemic foods you can expect your child to do the same.
- Do clear out junk food from your house. No child will learn to eat well if there is sweet temptation all around.
- Do set up a star chart for fruit and vegetables with a star for every serving. Aim for five or six stars. A child who fills up with healthy snacks is less likely to go for fattening ones.
- Do make exercise a part of family life – turn off the TV or computer or playstation and encourage active unstructured play to keep children active.

Don'ts:

- Don't insist your children finish all their food.
- Don't give children food as a way to keep them occupied. Give them something to play with instead.
- Don't give your children food during the day or night to comfort them.
- Don't underestimate the importance of sleep. Lack of sleep can upset blood sugar balance and stimulate appetite.
- Don't forget snacks. Children need regular nibbles to keep their blood sugar levels steady and to prevent cravings and bingeing on unhealthy food. Good ideas are seeds, cheese, sugarless cereal, fruit, raw veggies, sandwiches and yogurt.
- Don't be tempted to give children under 5 low fat milk, dairy produce or foods. Young children rely on a certain amount of fat as a source of calories and should not be placed on a low fat diet. This age group needs healthy fats for growth – but keep portion sizes small.

Age 6 to 11

It's normal at this age for fat to accumulate on the tummy and trunk until adolescence; on average children gain about 2 to 3kg (5 to 7lb) between the ages of 6 and 10. Expect children to put on weight before a major growth spurt. They fill out, then shoot up.

Dos:

- Do start teaching your child the basics of healthy eating and warn him or her about the dangers of being overweight.
- Do encourage your children to help you with the preparation and selection of food. Allow them to serve themselves and stop eating when they are full.
- Do eat the same food as your children do, and make family mealtimes a happy time.
- Do set up a healthy snack shelf in your cupboard.
- Do encourage your child to eat 3–6 servings a day of whole grains and anything made from them; 2–4 servings a day of fruit, 3–5 servings a day of vegetables and legumes and 2–3 servings of low fat dairy products and milk.
- Do enrol children in regular sports activities and take an interest in their progress.
- Do set time limits for television and computer work.

Don'ts:

- Don't give children sweet or fizzy drinks, as research[60] suggests that children who eat more sweetened beverages tend to have a higher risk of obesity.
- Don't underestimate the importance of body image if your child is overweight; she may be teased or bullied at school. Make sure she feels positive about her body.
- Don't give unlimited pocket money. Consumption of sweets and crisps on the way to school is a major cause of obesity.

Age 12 to 18

It's normal during the adolescent growth spurt for boys to gain more fat on their trunks while fat on their arms and legs decreases. In contrast, girls gain weight everywhere during this period. Girls may put on about 7kg (15lb) or more in body weight and boys during their peak growth period gain an average of 14kg (31lb).

Dos:

- Do continue to offer healthy meals, even if they are snubbed. Offer fruit when a hungry teenager returns from school and healthy snacks for breaks, and ban eating in front of the television.
- Teens can be lazy, so strike a deal with them and encourage them to get at least an hour of exercise or physical activity a day. Send teens on errands and involve them in household chores – anything that keeps them away from the television and computer.
- Do offer incentives for healthy eating and exercise – extra pocket money usually succeeds! Encourage your child to use the money for hobbies and interests and not food.
- Even if they don't appear to be listening, make sure you teach teens the basics of healthy eating. Explain that we are what we eat and how healthy eating and regular exercise will help them look and feel good and improve memory and concentration for school.
- Do encourage your child to wear trendy clothes and take pride in his or her appearance.

Don'ts:

- Don't underestimate the importance of peer pressure. Teens like to fit in, not stand out, so you need to negotiate a healthy balance between the junk food culture and healthy eating. If all your teenager's friends have sweet snacks, offer low fat, low glycaemic varieties such as bananas, dried apricots or dark chocolate.
- Don't put your child on a diet. The teenage years are a period of intense growth and development and teenagers need plenty of nutritious food to grow into their natural body weight.
- Don't force the issue. If your teenager is overweight he or she will undoubtedly feel embarrassed, and drawing attention to it will make things worse. It's better to change the whole family's eating habits and choice of leisure activity, so that healthier options become a way of life.

10

Glycaemic factor guidelines for eating out

Eating out on a glycaemic factor diet isn't a problem. The essential ingredients of glycaemic factor eating are the same foods that make up most restaurant meals – meats, fish, poultry, vegetables and fruits – and you should be able to find low glycaemic factor dishes in almost every restaurant. You may have to ask the waiter to make a few changes to your selected dish, for example to skip the sauce or to exchange the chips for a side salad, but most restaurants will do that. You shouldn't feel uncomfortable asking for changes to be made – remember, the restaurant is there to meet your needs, not the other way round.

It's important not to feel really hungry when you go out as this will just make you eat more, so ensure that you don't skip meals earlier in the day. It's also a good idea to drink a large glass of water before going out as thirst is often confused with hunger. When you arrive at the restaurant, remind yourself to focus on the celebration and the people you are with rather than the food, or if you are dining alone, the book or magazine you have brought to read. Your aim is to leave the restaurant feeling pleasantly full, not stuffed!

There are a vast number of places where you can eat out these days so here are some general guidelines, followed by specific advice on what to order at different kinds of restaurants.

- Unless you are eating at an exclusive and expensive restaurant, most restaurant portions are huge – big enough for two or three people. If that's the case, share your entrée and your meal with a friend. Just ask your waiter to bring an extra plate.
- You don't need to restrict high glycaemic factor food choices completely – remember the 80–20 rule – as long as the majority of foods on your plate are low glycaemic factor the overall glycaemic factor will still be fairly low.
- As mentioned above, don't be shy about asking for changes to be made in the way your dish is prepared or served.
- Skip the bread basket.
- Lean meat or fish with vegetables and salads are always superb choices.
- Be careful with the sauces you are offered – plain tomato or

cheese is usually best. If you aren't sure, skip the sauce and ask for extra vegetables instead.

- Exchange chips or potatoes with vegetables or a side salad.
- If the main course doesn't appeal, order two starters instead.
- As you look at your plate, think half vegetables, quarter protein and quarter low glycaemic factor carbohydrates and you should be fine.
- When it comes to dessert avoid high sugar pastries and cakes. Fresh fruit is always your best choice. You could also go for a small amount of ice cream or cheese with grapes or celery, but no biscuits.
- If you feel confused by the menu or can't translate the foreign names used for dishes on the menu, ask your waiter to explain and/or interpret.

British

Stick with foods that have been simply cooked and you should be okay.

Avoid full English breakfast with fried bread, side orders of bread and rolls, pastries, meat, potato and fish pies, battered or crumbed fish, Yorkshire pudding, chips, anything fried, mashed potato, traditional puddings such as Spotted Dick and custard, and beer.

Go for porridge and oatcakes, wholemeal bread or toast, grilled or poached fish and eggs, Dover sole, grilled lean meat, grilled liver and bacon and simple beef, game or pork roasts with no crackling.

Chinese

Avoid any white rice. It is almost always the short grain sticky variety which has a high glycaemic factor. Noodles aren't much better. Also avoid sesame prawn toasts, dim sum, spring rolls, sweet and sour dishes and toffee apples or bananas. And try to eat in a restaurant that doesn't use monosodium glutamate (MSG) for flavouring as it has a high glycaemic factor.

Go for clear soups, stir-fried vegetables, baked and grilled fish, stir-fried beef or chicken but no thick sauce, boiled (not fried) cellophane noodles which have been made from mung beans, dishes made from tofu (bean curd), and savoury dishes such as soy, ginger and garlic. Crispy duck is fine as long as you skip the sauce and hold back on the pancakes. Beef with Chinese mushrooms, prawn platter and chicken or pork with walnuts, sweetcorn or cashew nuts are all okay too.

French

The main things to avoid here are the cream sauces, pastries and tarts. So steer clear of creamy soups and sauces, pastry, potatoes, chips, quiches, crepes and profiteroles. Go for French onion soup, without the toast and cheese, salads with oily fish such as nicoise, cassoulet (meat and bean casserole), mussels in wine and onion sauce, crudités and grilled steak or fish.

Greek

The Greeks use olive oil and lemon and a variety of herbs and spices to cook and flavour their meals, so if you choose carefully you can enjoy a fine meal. Avoid rice with stuffed vine leaves, moussaka, pastry dishes, calamari, breads and meat balls and sausages. Go for Greek salad with feta cheese and a small wholewheat pitta bread, hummus and taramasalata with vegetable dips, bean casseroles, stews and soups, meat and vegetable kebabs, grilled fish, grilled seafood and meat casseroles.

Indian

Most Indian restaurants have a great selection of vegetable and legume dishes which are usually low glycaemic factor. Avoid breads (naan, chapattis, puri, roti, poppadums), deep-fried appetizers with batter or pastry, rice dishes, potato dishes, dishes with coconut and all Indian desserts. Go for tandoori and balti dishes with salad or basmati rice, baked or grilled meat dishes, vegetable dishes, dahl (lentil dishes), chana (chickpea dishes), fresh guava and raita, a delicious cucumber and yogurt dip.

Italian

Pasta and pizza tend to spring to mind when Italian restaurants are mentioned but there are plenty of other ways to enjoy Italian cuisine. Avoid garlic bread and breadsticks, egg pasta with creamy sauces, risottos, polenta, deep pan or medium pan pizzas, meat cooked in breadcrumbs and desserts like tiramisu and panna cotta. Go for thin soups, tuna nicoise salad, tricolour salad, seafood salads, carpaccio, antipasti which is a selection of grilled vegetables and lean meats, grilled fish, chicken or veal, one slice of thin-based pizza with vegetable or tomato and onion topping, a small portion of pasta (not egg pasta) with vegetable sauce and no grated cheese, and fresh fruits for dessert.

Japanese

Sushi isn't a great choice on a glycaemic factor diet because of the rice content. Sashami, however, is a good choice. Avoid rice, potatoes and noodles, apart from cellophane noodles, vegetables that have been deep fried, anything coated in breadcrumbs and fried, anything in rice wrappers and anything with miso (fermented beans) and mirin (sweetened sake). Instead choose green vegetables like spinach or beans or shiitake mushrooms, tofu dishes, mixed fish casseroles, steamed fish or chicken, soy bean casserole and meat and vegetables with tofu or cooked in a stock pot on your table.

Mexican

Beans are used in Mexican soups and dishes but avoid refried beans (frijoles refritos) that have been cooked in oil. Avoid any dish made with tortillas, nachos, tacos, burritos, enchiladas, quesadillas and chimichangas. It's also best to stay away from Mexican filled rolls and sandwiches, rice dishes, thick rich sauces and pastries and desserts. Go for guacamole dip with vegetables, raw fish salad with avocado, black bean soup, cold beef salad, chilli con carne with no rice, grilled fish, chicken or meat and salsas.

Middle Eastern

Low glycaemic factor nuts, beans and lentils are often used as an ingredient. Side salads and grilled meats and fish are also frequently available. Avoid couscous, tabbouleh, vine leaves, potato dishes, savoury pastries, honey pastries and all cakes. Instead go for falafel (rissoles made with chickpeas), hummus, kebabs without bread or rice, meatballs cooked on skewers, bean salad and baba ghanoush (grilled and pureed aubergine with tahine and lemon).

Spanish tapas bar

Avoid paella, the classic rice-based Spanish dish, and any other rice or potato-based dishes. It's also best to steer clear of churros (deep-fried strips of sweet batter), Spanish omelette and flan. Instead go for anchovies in vinegar, olives and nuts, grilled meats and salad, pickled chillies, gazpacho but without croutons, grilled fish and seafood and *pollo en pepitoria* (chicken braised with almonds).

Thai

Avoid rice and coconut rice-based dishes, spring rolls, fried or crispy noodles and soups made with rice or noodles. Go for prawn and papaya salad; mango and salmon soup; clear soups with chicken, fish or vegetables; satay with chicken, meat and a small amount of peanut sauce; steamed mussels with basil; curries but without the rice; beef or chicken salads; steamed tofu dishes; cellophane noodles made from mung beans; and tropical fruits.

Fast food

Fast food is always going to be high on the glycaemic factor but there are ways around it. Here are some ideas:

- If you get a burger in a bun, exchange the bun for a salad.
- If possible exchange the breaded deep-fried meat or fish for non-breaded meat or fish, but if you can't do that just scrape off the batter and breadcrumbs and eat what you find inside.
- Avoid chips and tomato ketchup.
- If you order a sandwich discard the top and eat it open.
- Order a salad but limit the amount of croutons and extras you eat and pass on the fatty dressings and sauces you'll be offered.
- If you must have a full English breakfast or fry up, it's best to stick with eggs, bacon, tomato, sausage and mushroom and to skip the fried bread.
- If you order a coffee ask for a plain coffee with milk or pouring cream or whipped cream. Coffee has no carbohydrates and a hint of cream now and again is fine as it will be lower in calories and GI than a latte.
- Avoid sugary and fizzy drinks and go for water or herbal tea instead.
- Never supersize anything.
- If you order a pizza, peel off the topping and eat it. Toss out the crust.

Packed lunch

For picnics and packed lunches don't be tempted to throw in sweets, crisps, fizzy rinks, sweet biscuits and cakes or anything fried. There are plenty of low glycaemic factor options to choose from.

- For sandwiches choose bread that is high in fibre such as wholegrain or granary bread or try wholemeal pitta, linseed rye bread, oatcakes, rye crispbreads or pumpernickel. Low glycaemic sandwich fillings include prepared salad vegetables such as cucumber, lettuce and tomatoes, low fat cottage cheese, lean cooked skinless chicken, canned oily fish, smoked mackerel pâté, lean roast beef or ham, taramasalata and nut butter.
- For packed salads good choices would be grilled Mediterranean vegetables with olive oil and balsamic vinegar or beansprouts, chickpeas, spring onion and watercress with a ginger and soy dressing. You could also go for raw vegetable crudités such as carrots, celery and cauliflower with a dip such as hummus. Peas with lean ham make a tasty snack, as does cooked pearl barley with radishes, spring onions, avocado, pumpkin seeds, crumbled feta cheese and dried fruit. Tuna and egg nicoise or goat's cheese on rocket salad with tomatoes or mixed bean salad are also fine choices.
- Be sure to bring plenty of fruits such as cherries, raspberries, figs, peaches, pears, grapes, tangerines, oranges and apples. Oaten biscuits, unsalted nuts, seeds, dried fruit and olives are also good for snacks.
- For drinks you could take soup, fruit smoothies or herbal teas in a flask, but the ideal and easiest choice is water.
- The best food choices at a party buffet are meat and fish that isn't breaded or battered, salads, quiche if you cut off the pastry, sausage rolls if you cut off the pastry, Caesar salad, coleslaw, cheeses, prawn cocktail, smoked salmon, three or four new potatoes and olive oil-based dressings. Avoid garlic bread, pasta salad, rice salad and sandwiches and rolls that aren't wholegrain.

Eating at parties or at a friend's home or at restaurants isn't really about the food, it's about the occasion, friendship and good times. Don't let food get in the way of that. Plan ahead, choose your food wisely, enjoy eating your food and make the most of the people you are with.

Conclusion: The glycaemic factor golden rules

1 Eat three meals a day and at least two snacks. Never skip meals, especially breakfast.
2 When you eat meals, how much you are eating is as important as what you are eating. Don't supersize anything. A good rule of thumb is not to eat more than you could fit into your cupped hands. Your aim is to feel satisfied at the end of your meal, not stuffed and bloated.
3 Always ensure your meals have a proper balance of low glycaemic carbohydrates, protein and heart-healthy fat. A simple rule to remember is when you look at your dinner plate, around half should be filled with vegetables, a quarter with protein – such as legumes, nuts, seeds and low fat dairy – and a quarter with healthy carbohydrates, such as whole grains, cereals, pasta, rice and potatoes. This is the essence of a healthy meal.
4 A good way to increase your chances of getting all the nutrients you need for good health is to make sure the portions of vegetables and fruits you eat in a day are different colours: dark green spinach, yellow corn, red peppers, orange carrots, black-berries and so on. Make sure your plate is filled with the natural colours of fresh food and you will be getting your nutrients.
5 Another way to ensure you are eating healthily is to eat as many foods as you can that are fresh and pure. 'Fresh' generally refers to food that doesn't come in a can or box. 'Pure' means nothing artificial and nothing added, including poisons, pesticides or – one of the biggest culprits – refined carbohydrates, commonly called sugar.
6 Drink plenty of fluids, especially water.
7 When you do eat food that has a high glycaemic factor, watch your portion size and accompany it with at least two low glycaemic factor foods of the same or larger quantity.
8 If the meal allows, add something acidic. Acid integrated into a food slows its conversion to glucose. This means eating half a grapefruit with breakfast, accompanying a pasta meal with a side salad topped with vinegar or lemon juice. You could even try drinking a glass of hot water with a squeeze of lemon or lime

juice in it, as the acid factor will reduce the GI of some high sugar foods by 30 per cent.

9 The aim is to keep your total GL per day under 100, under 75 if you want to lose weight.

10 Move about more. Exercise for 30 minutes a day or 10 minutes three times a day. Take the stairs instead of the lift.

11 Set attainable goals if you want to lose weight. Try to lose around half a kilo (1lb) a week and record and celebrate your progress.

12 Cooking can alter the GI value of food. The longer something is cooked the less nutrients and fibre will remain. Lightly steaming or eating vegetables raw makes your digestive system work harder and lowers the GI value of the meal.

13 Remember the 80–20 rule. Eat healthily 80 per cent of the time and you can afford the occasional indulgence. On a glycaemic factor diet no food is off limits.

14 Don't think of the glycaemic factor as a diet. It's a healthy eating programme that will last you for the rest of your life.

Useful addresses

British Dietetic Association
Fifth Floor, Charles House
148–149 Great Charles Street
Queensway
Birmingham B3 3HT
Tel.: 0121 200 8080
Website: www.bda.uk.com
Email: info@bda.uk.com

British Heart Foundation
14 Fitzhardinge Street
London W1H 6DH
Tel.: 020 7935 0185
Heart Info Line: 08450 70 80 70
Website: www.bhf.org.uk
Email: internet@bhf.org.uk

British Nutrition Foundation
High Holborn House
52–54 High Holborn
London WC1V 6RQ
Tel.: 020 7404 6504
Website: www.nutrition.org
Email: postbox@nutrition.org.uk

Coronary Prevention Group
2 Taviton Street
London WC1H 0BT
Tel.: 020 7927 2125 (9 a.m. to 5 p.m., Monday to Friday)
Website: www.healthnet.org.uk

Diabetes UK
10 Parkway
London NW1 7AA
Careline: 0845 120 2960
Website: www.diabetes.org.uk
Email: info@diabetes.org.uk

Institute for Optimum Nutrition
13 Blades Court
Deodar Road
London SW15 2NU
Tel.: 0870 979 1122 (9 a.m. to 5 p.m., Monday to Friday)
Website: www.ion.ac.uk

Useful websites

A *Glycaemic factor lists*

www.mendosa.com
A terrific and helpful website which includes information on the glycaemic index and load of every food tested. The latest books on the glycaemic index are reviewed, too.

www.glycaemicindex.com
Website sponsored by the University of Sydney in Australia that contains useful information on the glycaemic index and the glycaemic index of various carbohydrates. The website contains information from the glycaemic index expert Jennie Brand-Miller.

www.dietfreedom.co.uk
Information about and listings for the glycaemic load by Nigel Denby, author of *The GL Diet: Diet Freedom.*

www.gidiet.com
Information about the glycaemic index by Rick Gallop, author of *The GI Diet.*

Other useful websites

www.bodyfoods.com
www.waitrose.com/food_drink/nutrition/healthy
www.sainsburys.com/healthyeating
www.ivillage.co.uk (Tesco diet queries)
www.asda.com
www.womens-health-concern.org (Women's Health Concern)
www.hsph.harvard.edu/nutritionsource/ (Solid information about nutrition, weight and fitness)
www.mayohealth.org. (Search for answers to your questions about the glycaemic index from the Mayo clinic health and nutrition experts)
www.hlm.nih.gov/medlineplus/childnutrition.html (Medline's portal for advice about good nutrition for children of all ages)

116

www.nnh.org/products/gnsf.htm (Good nutrition for seniors from
the American National Network for Health)

Further reading

Beale, Lucy and Clarke, Joan, *The Complete Idiot's Guide to Glycemic Index Weight Loss*. Alpha Books, East Rutherford, NJ, 2005.

Brand-Miller, Jennie, *The Low GI Diet*. Hodder, London, 2005.

Brand-Miller, Jennie, *The New Glucose Revolution*. Marlowe, New York, 2004.

Denby, Nigel, *The GL Diet: Diet Freedom*. Blake, London, 2005.

Foster, Helen, *Easy GI Diet*. Hamlyn, London, 2004.

Gallop, Rick, *The GI Diet*. Virgin, London, 2003.

Govindji, Azmina, and Puddefoot, Nina, *The GI Plan*. Vermillion, London, 2004.

Holford, Patrick, *Patrick Holford's New Optimum Nutrition Bible*. Piatkus, London, 2004.

McKeith, Gillian, *You Are What You Eat*. Penguin, London, 2004.

Worrall Thompson, Antony, *Antony Worrall Thompson's GI Diet*. Kyle Cathie Ltd, London, 2005.

Notes

1 D.W. Ludvig et al. (2002) 'The glycaemic index: physiological mechanisms relating to obesity, diabetes, and cardiovascular disease', *Journal of the American Medical Association*, 8 May, 287(18): 2414–23.

2 L.S. Augustin et al. (2002) 'Glycaemic index in chronic disease: a review', *European Journal of Clinical Nutrition*, November, 56(11): 1049–71.

3 J. Brand-Miller (2003) 'Glycaemic load and chronic disease', *Nutrition Review*, May, 61(5 Pt 2): S49–55.

4 P. Westerterp et al. (2004) 'Fat intake and energy-balance effects', *Physiological Behaviour*, 30 December, 83(4): 579–85.

5 D. Schoeller et al. (2005) 'Energetics of obesity and weight control: does diet composition matter?' *Journal of the American Dietary Association (JAMA)*, May, 105(5 Suppl. 1): S24–8.

6 S.J. Bell et al. (2003) 'Low-glycaemic-load diets: impact on obesity and chronic diseases', *Critical Review of Food Science and Nutrition*, 43(4): 357–77.

7 S. Arora et al. (2005) 'The case for low carbohydrate diets in diabetes management', *Nutrition and Metabolism* (London), 14 July, 2(1): 16.

8 M. Pereira et al. (2004) 'Effects of a low-glycaemic load diet on resting energy expenditure and heart disease risk factors during weight loss', *JAMA*, 24 November, 292(20): 2482–90.

9 S. Liu et al. (2001) 'Dietary carbohydrates, physical inactivity, obesity, and the "metabolic syndrome" as predictors of coronary heart disease', *Current Opinion in Lipidology*, August, 12(4): 395–404.

10 P. Columbani et al. (2004) 'Glycaemic index and load-dynamic dietary guidelines in the context of diseases', *Physiological Behaviour*, 30 December, 83(4): 603–10.

11 M. Pereira et al. (2004) 'Effects of a low-glycaemic load diet on resting energy expenditure and heart disease risk factors during weight loss', *JAMA*, 24 November, 292(20): 2482–90; S. Bell et al. (2003) 'Low-glycaemic-load diets: impact on obesity and chronic diseases', *Critical Review of Food Science and Nutrition*, 43(4): 357–77.

12 C. Mobbs et al. (2005) 'Impaired glucose signaling as a cause of obesity and the metabolic syndrome: the glucoadipostatic hypothesis', *Physiological Behaviour*, 19 May 85(1): 3–23.

13 M. Harber et al. (2005) 'Effects of dietary carbohydrate restriction with high protein intake on protein metabolism and the somatotropic axis', *Journal of Clinical Endocrinology and Metabolism*, 21 June, 90; A. Astrup et al. (2005) 'The role of dietary fat in obesity', *Seminars in Vascular Medicine*, February, 5(1): 40–7.

14 J. Salmermon et al. (1997) 'Dietary fibre, glycaemic load, and risk of non-insulin-dependent diabetes mellitus in women', *JAMA*, 12 February, 277(6): 472–7.

15 F. Pasanisi et al. (2001) 'Benefits of sustained moderate weight loss in obesity', *Nutrition, Metabolism and Cardiovascular Diseases*, December, 11(6): 401–6.

16 A. Renko et al. (2005) 'The relationship of glucose tolerance to sleep disorders and daytime sleepiness', *Diabetes Research and Clinical Practice*, January, 67(1): 84–91.

17 S. Patel et al. (2004) 'A prospective study of sleep duration and mortality risk in women', *Sleep*, 1 May, 27(3): 440–4.

18 E. Ostman et al. (2005) 'Vinegar supplementation lowers glucose and insulin responses and increases satiety after a bread meal in healthy subjects', *European Journal of Clinical Nutrition*, September, 59(9): 983–8.

19 J. McMillan et al. (2004) 'Dietary approaches to overweight and obesity', *Clinical Dermatology*, July–August, 22(4): 310–4; C. Ebbeling et al. (2003) 'A reduced-glycaemic load diet in the treatment of adolescent obesity', *Archives of Pediatric Adolescent Medicine*, August, 157(8): 773–9; M. Pereira et al. (2004) 'Effects of a low-glycaemic load diet on resting energy expenditure and heart disease risk factors during weight loss', *JAMA*, 24 November, 292(20): 2482–90.

20 S. Bell et al. (2003) 'Low-glycaemic-load diets: impact on obesity and chronic diseases', *Critical Review of Food Science and Nutrition*, 43(4): 357–77.

21 D. Hensrud et al. (2004) 'Diet and obesity', *Current Opinions in Gastroenterology*, March; 20(2): 119–24.

22 C. Strik et al. (2005) 'The role of a low-glycaemic-index diet in the management of obesity', *American Journal of Clinical Nutrition*, April, 81(4): 940–1; J. McMillan et al. (2004) 'Dietary approaches to overweight and obesity', *Clinical Dermatology*, July–August, 22(4): 310–14.

23 M. Jacobson et al. (2004) 'Impact of improved glycaemic control on quality of life in patients with diabetes', *Endocrinology Practice*, November–December, 10(6): 502–8.

24 A. Hodge et al. (2004) 'Glycaemic index and dietary fibre and the risk of type 2 diabetes', *Diabetes Care*, November, 27(11): 2701–6.

25 V. Lewis et al. (2005) 'Prevention of coronary heart disease: a nonhormonal approach', *Seminars in Reproductive Medicine*, May, 23(2): 157–66.

26 M. Pereira et al. (2004) 'Effects of a low-glycaemic load diet on resting energy expenditure and heart disease risk factors during weight loss', *JAMA*, 24 November, 292(20): 2482–90.

27 A. Leeds et al. (2002) 'Glycaemic index and heart disease', *American Journal of Clinical Nutrition*, July, 76(1): 286S–9S; B. Schneeman et al. (2001) 'Use of glycaemic index in predicting risk of coronary heart disease', *American Journal of Clinical Nutrition*, January, 73(1): 130–1; J. Brand-Miller et al. (2004) 'Glycaemic index in relation to coronary disease', *Asia Pacific Journal of Clinical Nutrition*, 13(Suppl): S3.

28 F. Hu et al. (2002) 'Optimal diets for prevention of coronary heart disease', *JAMA*, 27 November, 288(20): 2569–78.

29 J. Sun et al. (2001) 'Hyperinsulinemia and insulin resistance related metabolic syndrome', *Chang Gung Medical Journal*, January, 24(1): 11–18.

30 D. Michaud et al. (2005) 'Dietary glycaemic load, carbohydrate, sugar, and colorectal cancer risk in men and women', *Cancer Epidemiology Biomarkers and Prevention*, January, 14(1): 138–47; S. Silvera et al. (2005) 'Dietary carbohydrates and breast cancer risk: a prospective study of the roles of overall glycaemic index and glycaemic load', *International Journal of Cancer*, 20 April, 114(4): 653–8; L. Augustin et al. (2004) 'Glycaemic index, glycaemic load and risk of gastric cancer', *Annals of Oncology*, April, 15(4): 581–4; D. Michaud et al. (2002) 'Dietary sugar, glycaemic load, and pancreatic cancer risk in a prospective study', *Journal of the National Cancer Institute*, 4 September, 94(17): 1293–300; J. Brand-Miller et al. (2003) 'Glycaemic load and chronic disease', *Nutrition Review*, May, 61(5 Pt 2): S49–55; L. Augustin et al. (2003) 'Dietary glycaemic index, glycaemic load and ovarian cancer risk: a case-control study in Italy', *Annals of Oncology*, January, 14(1): 78–84; L. Augustin et al. (2003) 'Glycaemic index and glycaemic load

in endometrial cancer', *International Journal of Cancer*, 20 June, 105(3): 404–7.

31 D. Jenkin et al. (2002) 'Glycaemic index: overview of implications in health and disease', *American Journal of Clinical Nutrition*, July, 76(1): 266S–73S.

32 A. Rossignol et al. (1991) 'Prevalence and severity of the premenstrual syndrome. Effects of foods and beverages that are sweet or high in sugar content', *Journal of Reproductive Medicine*, February, 36(2): 131–6; K. Trout et al. (2004) 'Insulin sensitivity and premenstrual syndrome', *Current Diabetes Reports*, August, 4(4): 273–80.

33 A. Tollino et al. (2005) 'Evaluation of ovarian functionality after a dietary treatment in obese women with polycystic ovary syndrome', *European Journal of Obstetrics and Gynaecology and Reproductive Biology*, 1 March, 119(1): 87–93.

34 S. Rice et al. (2005) 'Impaired insulin-dependent glucose metabolism in granulosa-lutein cells from anovulatory women with polycystic ovaries', *Human Reproduction*, February, 20(2): 373–81 (e-pub. 11 November 2004).

35 A. Moran et al. (2004) 'Understanding and managing disturbances in insulin metabolism and body weight in women with polycystic ovary syndrome', *Best Practice and Research Clinical Obstetrics and Gynaecology*, October, 18(5): 719–36.

36 S. Chow et al. (2005) 'Characteristics of glycaemic control in elite power and endurance athletes', *Preventative Medicine*, May, 40(5): 564–9.

37 L. Burke et al. (1998) 'Glycaemic index – a new tool in sport nutrition?' *International Journal of Sport Nutrition*, December, 8(4): 401–15.

38 C. Ebbeling et al. (2003) 'A reduced-glycaemic load diet in the treatment of adolescent obesity', *Archives of Pediatrics and Adolescent Medicine*, August, 157(8): 773–9.

39 K. Antshel et al. (2004) 'Cognitive strengths and weaknesses in children and adolescents homozygous for the galactosemia Q188R mutation: a descriptive study', *Neuropsychology*, October, 18(4): 658–64.

40 A. Convit, O.T. Wolf, C. Tarshish and M.J. De Leon (2003) 'Reduced glucose tolerance is associated with poor memory performance and hippocampal atrophy among normal elderly', *Proceedings of the National Academy of Science of the USA*, 18 February, 100(4): 2019–22.

41 P. Lustman et al. (2005) 'Depression in diabetic patients: the relationship between mood and glycaemic control', *Journal of Diabetes Complications*, March–April, 19(2): 113–22.

42 R. Deicher et al. (2005) 'Low total vitamin C plasma level is a risk factor for cardiovascular morbidity and mortality in hemodialysis patients', *Journal of the American Society of Nephrology*, June, 16(6): 1811–18 (e-pub. 6 April 2005).

43 D. Schaumberg et al. (2004) 'Dietary glycaemic load and risk of age-related cataract', *American Journal of Clinical Nutrition*, August, 80(2): 489–95.

44 L. Cordain et al. (2005) 'Origins and evolution of the Western diet: health implications for the 21st century', *American Journal of Clinical Nutrition*, February, 81(2): 341–54.

45 S. Scanto S. and J. Yudkin (1969) 'The effect of dietary sucrose on blood lipids, serum insulin, platelet adhesiveness and body weight in human volunteers', *Postgraduate Medicine Journal*, 45: 602–7; A. Sanchez et al. (1973) 'The role of sugars in human neutrophilic phagocytosis', *American Journal of Clinical Nutrition*, November, 261: 1180–4; J. Goldman et al. (1986) 'Behavioral effects of sucrose on preschool children', *Journal of Abnormal Child Psychology*, 14(4): 565–77; W. Ringsdorf, E. Cheraskin and R. Ramsay (1976) 'Sucrose, neutrophilic phagocytosis and resistance to disease', *Dental Survey*, 52(12): 46–8; J. Yudkin, S. Kang and K. Bruckdorfer (1960) 'Effects of high dietary sugar', *British Journal of Medicine*, 22 November, 281: 1396; A. Kozlovsky et al. (1966) 'Effects of diets high in simple sugars on urinary chromium losses', *Metabolism*, June, 35: 515–18; E. Takahashi (1982) 'Tohuku University School of Medicine', *Wholistic Health Digest*, October, 41; J. Kelsay et al. (1974) 'Diets high in glucose or sucrose and young women', *American Journal of Clinical Nutrition*, 27: 926–36; M. Fields et al. (1983) 'Effect of copper deficiency on metabolism and mortality in rats fed sucrose or starch diets', *Journal of Nutrition*, 113: 1335–45; J. Lemann (1967) 'Evidence that glucose ingestion inhibits net renal tubular reabsorption of calcium and magnesium', *Journal of Laboratory and Clinical Medicine*, 70: 236–45; H. Taub, ed., (1986) 'Sugar weakens eyesight', *VM Newsletter*, 6 May, 5; University of California, Berkeley (1989) *Wellness Letter*, December, 6(3): 4–5 (a quote from Dr Richard Wurtman, a neurobiologist at MIT); J. Lewis (1990) 'Health briefings', *Fort Worth Star Telegram*, 11 June (reported to the

NOTES

Society for Pediatric Research in Anaheim, CA, 9 May 1990 by
Dr Timothy Jones, a scientist from Perth, Australia); W.
Glinsmann, H. Irausquin and K. Youngmee (1986) *Evaluation of
Health Aspects of Sugars Contained in Carbohydrate Sweet-
eners. Report of Sugars Task Force* (Washington, DC: Food and
Drug Administration), p. 39; H. Keen, B. Thomas, R. Jarrett and
J. Fuller (1979) 'Nutrient intake, adiposity, and diabetes', *British
Medical Journal*, 1: 655–8; L. Darlington et al. (1986) 'Placebo-
controlled, blind study of dietary manipulation therapy in
rheumatoid arthritis', *Lancet*, 1: 6 February: 236–8; K. Heaton
(1984) 'The sweet road to gallstones', *British Medical Journal*,
14 April, 288: 1103–4; J. Yudkin (1964) 'Dietary fat and dietary
sugar in relation to ischemic heart disease and diabetes', *Lancet*,
2: 4; T. Cleave and G. Campbell (1960) *Diabetes, Coronary
Thrombosis and the Saccharine Disease* (Bristol: John Wright);
K. Behall (1982) 'Influence of oestrogen content of oral
contraceptives and consumption of sucrose on blood para-
meters', *Diss. Abstr. Int. B*, 43: 1437; H. Beck-Nielsen, O.
Pedersen and N.S. Sorensen (1978) 'Effects of diet on the
cellular insulin binding and the insulin sensitivity in young
healthy subjects', *Diabetes*, 15: 289–96; H. Keen, B. Thomas, R.
Jarrett and J. Fuller (1977) 'Nutritional factors in diabetes
mellitus', in J. Yudkin, ed., *Diet of Man: Needs and Wants*,
London: Applied Science, pp. 89–108; L. Gardner and S. Reiser
(1982) 'Effects of dietary carbohydrates on fasting levels of
human growth hormone and cortisol', *Proceedings of the Society
of Experimental Biological Medicine*, 169: 36–40; S. Reiser
(1985) 'Effects of dietary sugars on metabolic risk factors
associated with heart disease', *Nutritional Health*, 3: 203–16; R.
Hodges T. and Rebello (1983) 'Carbohydrates and blood
pressure', *Annals of Internal Medicine*, 98: 838–41; D. Behar, J.
Rapoport, J. Adams, C. Berg and M. Cornblath (1984) 'Sugar
challenge testing with children considered behaviorally sugar
reactive', *Nutritional Behavior*, 1: 277–88; E. Grand (1979)
'Food allergies and migraine', *Lancet*, 1: 955–9; no author
(1974) 'Sucrose induces diabetes in cat', *Federal Protocol*, 6:
97; P. Moynihan et al. (2004) 'Diet, nutrition and the prevention
of dental diseases', *Public Health and Nutrition*, February,
7(1A): 201–26; S. Vermunt et al. (2003) 'Effects of sugar intake
on body weight: a review', *Obesity Review*, May, 4(2): 91–9; L.
Peters et al. (2003) 'Effects of high sucrose diet on body and

124

liver weight and hepatic enzyme content and activity in the rat', *In Vivo*, January–February, 17(1): 61–5; D. Michaud et al. (2002) 'Dietary sugar, glycaemic load, and pancreatic cancer risk in a prospective study', *Journal of the National Cancer Institute*, 4 September, 94(17): 1293–300; M. Lean et al. (2004) 'Aspartame and its effects on health', *British Medical Journal*, 2 October, 329(7469): 755–6; M. Weihrauch et al. (2004) 'Artificial sweeteners – do they bear a carcinogenic risk?' *Annals of Oncology*, October, 15(10): 1460–5; T. Clausen et al. (2001) 'High intake of energy, sucrose, and polyunsaturated fatty acids is associated with increased risk of preeclampsia', *American Journal of Obstetrics and Gynecology*, August, 185(2): 451–8.

46 P. Columbani et al. (2004) 'Glycaemic index and load-dynamic dietary guidelines in the context of diseases', *Physiological Behaviour*, 30 December, 83(4): 603–10.

47 J. Brand-Miller (2003) 'Glycaemic load and chronic disease', *Nutrition Review*, May, 61(5 Pt 2): S49–55.

48 'Glycaemic load, diet, and health', *Harvard Women's Health Watch*, June (2001), 8(10): 1–2.

49 A. Flint et al. (2000) 'Reproducibility, power and validity of visual analogue scales in assessment of appetite sensations in single test meal studies', *International Journal of Obesity and Related Metabolic Disorders*, January, 24(1): 38–48.

50 S. Grantham et al. (2005) 'Can the provision of breakfast benefit school performance?' *Food Nutrition Bulletin*, June, 26(2 Suppl 2): S144–58.

51 E. Ostman et al. (2005) 'Vinegar supplementation lowers glucose and insulin responses and increases satiety after a bread meal in healthy subjects', *European Journal of Clinical Nutrition*, September, 59(9): 983–8.

52 A. Shalbert et al. (2005) 'Dietary polyphenols and the prevention of diseases', *Critical Review of Food Science and Nutrition*, 45(4): 287–306.

53 D. Hensurd et al. (2004) 'Diet and obesity', *Current Opinions in Gastroenterology*, March, 20(2): 119–24.

54 L. Serra et al. (2003–4) 'Mediterranean diet and health: is all the secret in olive oil?' *Pathophysiol Haemost Thromb.*, September 2003–December 2004, 33(5–6): 461–5.

55 M. Moyad et al. (2005) 'An introduction to dietary/supplemental omega-3 fatty acids for general health and prevention: part I', *Urological Oncology*, January–February, 23(1): 28–35.

56 M. Lean et al. (2004) 'Aspartame and its effects on health', *British Medical Journal*, 2 October, 329(7469): 755–6.
57 L. Robinson et al. (2004) 'Caffeine ingestion before an oral glucose tolerance test impairs blood glucose management in men with type 2 diabetes', *Journal of Nutrition*, October, 134(10): 2528–33.
58 L. Link et al. (2004) 'Raw versus cooked vegetables and cancer risk', *Cancer Epidemiological Biomarkers Preview*, September, 13(9); C. Brand et al. (1985) 'Food processing and the glycaemic index', *American Journal of Clinical Nutrition*, December, 42(6): 1192–6.
59 R. Mahoney et al. (2005) 'Effect of breakfast composition on cognitive processes in elementary school children', *Physiological Behaviour*, 5 August.
60 (2004) 'Soft drinks and obesity', *Journal of Pediatrics*, April, 144(4): 555–6.

Index

acidic foods 47, 112
ageing 59
American College of Sports
  Medicine 73–4
Atkins diet 1

beans and pulses 96
Beverly Hills diet 1–2
biscuits and crackers: ratings
  12
blood sugar levels: diabetes
  and insulin 51–2; keeping
  steady 8–9
body mass index 35, 41
Brand-Miller, Jennie: diet
  programme 33–5; *The
  Glucose Revolution: the
  Authoritative Guide to the
  Glycaemic Index* 3–4
breads 15, 17, 76; GI rating 11
breakfast 6, 91–2

calories 7
cancer 10, 54–5, 86
carbohydrates 78; beliefs about
  7; choices for GL 76–9;
  glycaemic load factor 27–30;
  other diet plans 1–2;
  shopping guidelines 95–6
cereals, breakfast 15, 17, 77,
  96; GI ratings 11–12
cereals and grains *see* grains
children: benefits of GI foods
  101–2; foods for age groups
  102–5; obesity in 57–8

cholesterol: good and bad fats
  86–7; types and effects of
  53
Conley, Rosemary 2

dairy products 17; low GL
  84–5; milk as a drink 90;
  ratings 12
Denby, Nigel 39
depression 86
diabetes: blood sugar levels
  8–10; GI diet for 2–3;
  obesity and 50; types and
  effects of 51–2 *see also*
  blood sugar levels; insulin
diet and nutrition 1–2; beliefs
  about 6–7; making healthy
  choices 30–1
drinks 16; alcoholic 90;
  glycaemic factor 89–90, 94,
  96–7; juices 24; ratings 14

emotions: depression 59;
  irritability 59; social factors
  111
exercise 113; 30 minutes a day
  45; aerobics, strength and
  flexibility 73–4; choosing
  and keeping a programme
  74–6; stress reduction 46–7

F-Plan diet 2
fats: beliefs about 6–7; cooking
  with 99; GI
  recommendations 19; good

127

polycystic ovary syndrome
(PCOS) 56–7
potatoes 15, 78
premenstrual syndrome (PMS)
55
proteins: GI recommendations
18–19; low GL 82–4; other
diet plans 1–2
Puddefoot, Nina 37–8

ratings 11–14
relaxation and rest 46–7
restaurants 106–10

salt 87
Scarsdale diet 1–2
Sear, Barry 40
seeds and nuts 96
snacks and sweets 16; beliefs
about 6; carbohydrates 78–9;
indulgences 46; ratings 14;
sugars and sweeteners 87–9
sport and physical performance

57
stress 46–7
sugar and sweeteners: types of
87–9
Syndrome X 53–4

thyroid function 50

vegetables 17, 97–8; cooking
99; low GL 80–2; ratings 14
vegetarians and vegans 83–4
vitamins and minerals:
recommendations 19–23;
supplementing with 47–8

water 46
weight: body mass index 41;
setting goals 40–2; stable
blood sugar and 32–3; waist
to hip ratio 41
Willett, Dr Walter 5, 26
Worrall Thompson, Antony 38